Trauma and Memory

T0383549

Trauma and Memory will assist mental health experts and professionals, as well as the interested public, in understanding the scientific issues around trauma memory, and how this differs from other areas of memory.

This book provides accounts of the damage caused to psychology and survivors internationally by false memory groups and ideas. It is unequivocally passionate about the truth of trauma memory and exposing the damaging disinformation that can seep into the field. Contributors to this book include leading professionals from the field of criminology, law, psychology and psychotherapy in the UK and USA, along with survivor-professionals who understand only too well the damage such disinformation can cause.

This book is a valuable resource for mental health professionals of all disciplines including those involved with relevant law and public health policy. It will also help survivors and survivor-professionals in gaining insight into the forces resisting disclosure.

Valerie Sinason, PhD, is a widely published Writer and Psychoanalyst. She has pioneered disability and trauma-informed therapy for over 30 years, is President of the Institute of Psychotherapy and Disability, Founder and Patron of the Clinic for Dissociative Studies and on the Board of the ISSTD.

Ashley Conway, PhD, AFBPsS, is a Counselling Psychologist. He has worked in a wide range of fields of trauma, ranging through severe critical incidents to long term abuse, and has published widely in these areas. He is currently the Chair of the Clinic for Dissociative Studies in London, UK.

Trauma and Memory

The Science and the Silenced

Edited by
Valerie Sinason and Ashley Conway

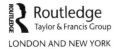
Routledge
Taylor & Francis Group

LONDON AND NEW YORK

First published 2022
by Routledge
2 Park Square, Milton Park, Abingdon, Oxon OX14 4RN

and by Routledge
605 Third Avenue, New York, NY 10158

Routledge is an imprint of the Taylor & Francis Group, an informa business

British Library Cataloguing in Publication Data
A catalogue record for this book is available from the British Library

Library of Congress Cataloging-in-Publication Data
A catalog record has been requested for this book

ISBN: 978-1-032-04432-3 (hbk)
ISBN: 978-1-032-04429-3 (pbk)
ISBN: 978-1-003-19315-9 (ebk)

DOI: 10.4324/9781003193159

Typeset in Times New Roman
by Taylor & Francis Books

We humbly dedicate this book to Professor Jennifer Freyd. We are in awe of her courage, dignity and her illuminating research lens, through which she has born her name and history.

The toxic international field of unscientific memory research and disinformation, with all its media backing, has its roots in an unprecedented attack on this one individual.

Her veracity, identity and professional credibility were publicly called into question. Through her dignity, resilience, hard work and brilliant research her name has been restored to her. She has been the antidote to the venom.

Valerie and Ashley

Contents

Tables

Editors

Ashley Conway is a psychologist with a long-term interest in trauma and memory. He is primarily a clinician, who is widely published. He has worked as a trauma consultant to the UK's Serious Organised Crime Agency and the United Nations. He has had a concerned interest in the development of the false memory syndrome (FMS) movement since its inception in the UK. He is currently Chair of the Clinic for Dissociative Studies in London.

Valerie Sinason is a poet, writer and retired child psychotherapist and adult psychoanalyst who has published over 17 books and 170 papers and chapters on disability, trauma and dissociation. She is President of the Institute for Psychotherapy and Disability (IPD) and Founder and Patron of the Clinic for Dissociative Studies. Her latest book "The Truth about trauma and dissociation, everything you didn't want to know and were afraid to ask" was published in 2020 and won the ISSTD Frank W Putnam award. Her first novel, "The Orpheus Project", will be published April 2022.

Contributors

Ruth Blizard, PhD, is an internationally known Psychologist practising for over 35 years in the USA. She has published articles integrating psychoanalytic concepts and attachment theory in the treatment of trauma, borderline personality, psychosis and the dissociative disorders. She is on the editorial board of the *Journal of Trauma and Dissociation*.

Winja Buss has worked in Youth Welfare for many years as well as being a researcher at the Trauma Institute, Leipzig. She has been widely published on trauma and dissociation in Europe as well as being on the Editorial Board of the ESTD Newsletter (European Society for Trauma and Dissociation), Board Member for the Psychotrauma Centre, Leipzig, and Secretary for the RAMCOA Special Interest Group of the ISSTD (International Society for the Study of Traumas and Dissociation).

Ross Cheit is a Professor of Political Science and International and Public Affairs at Brown University. As a law expert, he brings a fresh perspective to the memory debate. He draws on personal experience and years of research. He set up the hugely valuable online resource of the Recovered Memory Project and is the author of the highly influential book *The Witch Hunt Narrative*.

Lynn Crook, MEd, began investigating false memory claims following her successful recovered memory lawsuit in 1994. She has presented her findings at conferences in the US, Canada, Great Britain and at the United Nations. Her next book examines the successes and failures of the evolving false memory movement.

Jennifer Johns is a retired Fellow of the British Psychoanalytical Society. She was originally a GP, and has worked in the NHS as a psychotherapist in addition to practising psychoanalysis privately. She edited *The Ailment and Other Psychoanalytic Essays* (1989) by Tom Main, and was jointly editor of *Thinking about Children* by D.W. Winnicott (1996) and *Within Time and Beyond Time* (2001).

Brett Kahr is a Senior Fellow at the Tavistock Institute of Medical Psychology in London and, also, Visiting Professor of Psychoanalysis and Mental Health in the Regent's School of Psychotherapy and Psychology at Regent's University London. A Trustee of Freud Museum London and author of 15 books, he works with individuals and couples in Central London.

Phil Mollon is a Consultant Clinical Psychologist and Psychotherapist at Lister Hospital, Stevenage. He has written the book *Multiple Selves, Multiple Voices: Working with Trauma, Violation and Dissociation* (1998), and served on the British Psychological Society's Working Party on Recovered Memories.

Mary Sue Moore is a Consultant Clinical Psychologist and a licensed Child and Adult Psychotherapist in Boulder, Colorado, and an Honorary Senior Psychotherapist in the Child and Family Department at the Tavistock Clinic, London. She was awarded a Fulbright to work with John Bowlby in 1986–8 and worked with Bettelheim in 1977. She specialises in the analysis of children's drawings and the physiology and psychology of trauma, placing a special emphasis on attachment theory. Her book *Reflections of Self: The Impact of Trauma on Children's Drawings* will be published shortly.

Susie Orbach is a Psychotherapist, Psychoanalyst, Writer and Social Critic. She is the founder of the Women's Therapy Centre in London and the Women's Therapy Centre Institute, a postgraduate psychotherapy training centre in New York in 1981, a former *Guardian* columnist and Visiting Professor at the London School of Economics, and the author of many seminal books including *Hunger Strike, The Impossibility of Sex, Bodies, In Therapy* and the international bestseller *Fat is a Feminist Issue*. She lives in London and lectures extensively worldwide.

Marjorie Orr has an MA in Philosophy and English literature from Glasgow University and completed a Jungian psychotherapy training. She has been a features journalist and TV producer and continues to be a consulting media astrologer and novelist. This chapter came from her past work at Accuracy about Abuse, a leading international child abuse information service that she started and ran.

Khadija Rouf is a Consultant Clinical Psychologist and a member of the British Psychological Society's Safeguarding Advisory Group. Khadj has worked on resources for young people, and written professionally regarding mental health issues, both for clinicians and the public. She has also written personally from her perspective as a survivor of child abuse.

Mike Salter is a Senior Lecturer in criminology at Western Sydney University, where he leads the violence team of the Sexualities and Genders Research initiative. He is the author of two books published by Routledge (*Organised Sexual Abuse* and *Crime, Justice and Social Media*) and three dozen peer-reviewed papers and book chapters on abuse, trauma and violence. Dr Salter sits on the Board of Directors of the International Society for the Study of

Trauma and Dissociation and consults with a range of government and non-government agencies.

Ann Scott is a Senior Member of the British Psychotherapy Foundation (Psychoanalytic Psychotherapy Association) and a Training Therapist for the Independent Psychoanalytic Child and Adolescent Psychotherapy Association (BPF). She is Editor-in-Chief of the *British Journal of Psychotherapy*, and the literary executor of Isabel Menzies Lyth. She is the author, with the late Ruth First, of *Olive Schreiner: A Biography*; with the late Mary Barnes, of *Something Sacred: Conversations, Writings, Paintings;* and of *Real Events Revisited: Fantasy, Memory and Psychoanalysis.*

Danny Taggart is a Clinical Psychologist and Academic Director on the Doctorate in Clinical Psychology course at the University of Essex. He is an Honorary Clinical Psychologist in the Norfolk Parent Infant Mental Health service. He is currently seconded as Lead Clinician/Principal Psychologist at the Truth Project, part of the Independent Inquiry into Child Sexual Abuse (England and Wales).

Preface

This book, dedicated to my friend Jennifer Freyd, is a unique collection of perspectives on how society conspires, at various levels, to provide explanations that can be seized upon to provide a defence against allegations of abuse. For the abused, living as a child in an environment of inescapable trauma, compartmentalisation of the traumatic memories is a common and understandable survival technique. For reasons that become very clear by reading the reasoned contributions of this well-chosen set of accomplished authors, amnesias (and recovered memories) associated with child sexual abuse have become far more contentious than amnesias related to any other form of trauma.

Despite amnesias being included in the diagnostic criteria for post-traumatic stress disorder for decades, we have witnessed, beginning in the early 1990s, a backlash against belief in the accounts of individuals sexually abused as children. This was personified in the formal creation of the False Memory Syndrome Foundation in 1992 (and followed by the creation of other related organisations such as the British False Memory Society). At around the same time, we saw attempts to "create" false memories, such as those described in Elizabeth Loftus' "Lost in the Mall" study, to try and prove that recovered memories of abuse were legally unreliable.

A number of contributors to this volume bring the additional authenticity of having been abused themselves as children, and to have recovered memories of that abuse with subsequent legal judgements affirming the reality of what was done to them. They write with courage, clarity and authenticity.

The names that multiple contributors make reference to in this volume are sentinel figures in a debate that got underway in the late 19th century and which reached its polarising zenith in the "Memory Wars" of the 1990s. By 1994, 85% of the media coverage of adults' accusations of childhood sex abuse focused on false memories. There were serious attempts on the part of those allied with the FMSF to essentially ban therapy. Patients were encouraged to sue therapists. Therapists found themselves in court – where an adverse judgement would mean jail-time.

And then the fog began to clear.

Revelations in 2002 of the extent of child sexual abuse perpetrated by priests associated with the Boston archdiocese and the extent of the cover-up put beyond doubt that our most sacred institutions can sexually abuse children in extraordinary numbers. Why would that other societal institution, the family, be different? Then, numbers associated with child sex exploitation internet sites demonstrated the existence of verified child sexual abuse in industrial numbers. Prominent societal figures such as Jimmy Savile and Jerry Sandusky were exposed as prolific abusers. Societal movements that spoke out about abuse, such as the #MeToo movement, formed. Previously protected abusers such as Bill Cosby and Harvey Weinstein (notwithstanding an attempted "false memory" defence) found themselves in jail. This book chronicles and critiques the way we as a society have had to go to the brink, in order not to succumb to falsehood.

Professor Warwick Middleton MB BS, FRANZCP, MD
Professor, University of Queensland
Past President, International Society for the Study of Trauma & Dissociation
(ISSTD)

Acknowledgements

To our family, friends and colleagues for their love and support, and our patients who have privileged us with the beauty and courage of their narratives. Also, Kite Walker and to the memory of Cesare Sacerdoti. With special thanks to Sandy Dilip for bringing this book to birth, and to Routledge for taking it on.

Introduction

This book started life as a second edition to *Memory in Dispute* which was published in 1998. Since that time, some things have changed, and others sadly remain the same.

Much of the content of the original book, and indeed the additional insights in this book, relates to issues around the reliability of memory and the so-called "false memory syndrome" (FMS).

The American False Memory Syndrome Foundation (FMSF) was dissolved at the end of December 2019 just before this book went to press. Does this make the content any less relevant? We believe not. An organisation that has caused such grief to survivors, and the professionals who work with them, all over the world, has ended. Whilst this is a source of relief to those who care about a clinical and scientific understanding of trauma memory, the complex inheritance for victims and clinicians continues its toxic journey.

The FMS model provided an explanation for the beginning of the exposure of the scale of Child Sexual Abuse (CSA) worldwide, and it enabled the awful truth to be displaced. The multitude of stories of abuse that were beginning to be made public could be explained away – they could be blamed on the therapists who were hearing their clients' histories.

As long as truth struggles with power, there will be offshoots of such models of displacement and the history of denial goes far back. The FMS may have gone off-grid for now, but it is simply another move in the theories of denial of abuse, and more efforts to silence the truth will follow. The principles remain the same.

Sadly, the growing evidence from social media and the dark web has demonstrated that interest in the abuse of children has not gone away, and indeed may be worsening – both in terms of its extremity and the increasingly younger age of the victims. Over hundreds of years, society has found its way to deny the incidences and consequences of child sexual abuse. We believe that the so-called false memory syndrome is just another example of this, and that new examples will arise (e.g. the term "voluntary unwanted sex", which has recently been invented, creating confusion over what determines consent). Far from being less relevant now, we believe that there are very important lessons to be learnt from dealing with the last quarter-century of a pseudo-scientific model for the denial of reports of child sexual abuse.

DOI: 10.4324/9781003193159-1

Cassandra was a princess of Troy and a daughter of King Priam and Queen Hecuba. She was a priestess of Apollo and had taken a sacred vow of chastity to remain a virgin for life. What happened that led her to be seen as the prophetess who was destined never to be believed? Everything she correctly predicted and witnessed was denied and discredited. She was seen as insane for her prophecies. And hidden in this familiar attack on the testimony of a woman, however aristocratic, we find something chillingly familiar. Abuse.

She fought off Apollo when he tried to rape her, and as a punishment he condemned her to being disbelieved and discredited. Indeed, some sources, notably Aeschylus, tried to make her the perpetrator, saying she had promised sex to him and then refused him.

The account of Cassandra tragically fits Jennifer Freyd's concept of DARVO (Freyd, 1997). DARVO stands for Deny, Attack, and Reverse Victim and Offender. This is the common response of a person or an institution that will not accept responsibility and accountability for the violations they have caused.

The Cassandra myth is even more relevant at this historical moment when the American FMSF has finally dissolved, after spreading its anti-science around the world for nearly three decades. For long after the demise of the FMS Foundation, the notion of the invented diagnosis "false memory syndrome" will remain in psychology textbooks. Much of the FMS narrative was built upon the work of Elizabeth Loftus, and her famous "Lost in the Mall" study (Loftus & Pickrell, 1995). Yet very few have taken the time to actually read the original paper, realise how tiny the study was (24 subjects) or review its backstory. As Lynn Crook and Ruth Blizard demonstrate in their chapters in this book, that seminal paper, which became a cornerstone of the FMS narrative, is itself highly questionable.

The FMSF did not create the strategy of DARVO; it has been there since ancient times, as we can see from Cassandra. However, in our own historical period the practice of DARVO has garnered enormous media coverage, political acceptance and destroyed countless lives. The offshoots of the US FMSF will probably continue long after weaker templates dissolve. However, its deception in inventing a syndrome of "false memory", mixed with the societal fear of accepting the reality of the scale of CSA trauma made for a dangerous combination.

It is even more relevant when we consider the courage of Professor Jennifer Freyd. A key researcher in this field, she has had to bear the link of her name, with her parents who were the principal creators of the FMSF.

As human beings, our own narrative, our own story, is incredibly important. Except in a very few cases of distortion and fantasy (which can also be a consequence of trauma) our life stories are real. As a species it is how we communicate and learn from one another. It is part of the denying response to trauma that the word "story" has been contaminated and turned into fantasy or fiction, rather than being accepted as a precious possession we all have at the core of our identity.

Indeed, tellingly, in looking at the introduction of the 1998 book, there is only one sentence we would need to change – it is where the societal contamination affected one of us (Sinason, 1998) unknowingly, as if it came from a scientific consensus. "Individuals with severe dissociative disorders are particularly hypnotisable, suggestible and fantasy-prone, and they can enter auto-hypnotic trance states by themselves". Thanks to the seminal work of Simone Reinders (Reinders et al., 2012), we now know that individuals with Dissociative Identity Disorders are not more fantasy-prone than healthy control subjects.

The #MeToo movement has aided survivors and, in the UK, the impact of the enormity of abuse committed by Jimmy Savile has increased awareness significantly. However, the backlash is alive and well. With the curiously disproportionate imprisonment of Carl Beech in 2019 for 18 years for lying about his abuse at the hands of political VIPs (in the UK a sentence greater than for murder), already there has been a dramatic reduction in victims coming forward, and especially victims who allege abuse from well-known figures.

In the 1998 book, written at the height of the so-called "Memory Wars", there was an attempt at making a moral equivalence that was inaccurate. Now we can state with scientific confidence that in addition to ordinary memory that is never forgotten, recovered memories can indeed be real. Now there is a vast amount of evidence showing that people abused in childhood are able to "forget" the experience and subsequently recall it in later life. The line that the false memory groups have taken, that such things do not happen, is simply untrue. It is important to learn lessons from this experience, which has caused great harm to many victims of abuse.

Memory distortions happen, but naming the wrong person as an abuser is rare. But over the last 25 years such a narrative has received a vast amount of uncritical attention and belief in both the professional literature and popular press. This obsession with denying people's accounts of their abuse has received an enormously disproportionate amount of attention compared to the millions of people who struggle daily with dealing with the consequences of abuse in their adult life. There is a very important lesson here for clinicians, researchers, professional bodies and the legal system – to ask: what went wrong? How did such an inaccurate and harmful model come to be seen as scientific and solid?

Where the law is concerned, there is often one person's word against another's. Whilst assessment of individual cases might require the Judgement of Solomon, we nevertheless have evidence that over 8 million adults in the UK experienced abuse before the age of 16 (Office for National Statistics, 2020). Only a tiny percentage are considered to have falsified evidence. In other words, whilst every single case requires careful attention, as to be wrongly accused is also to be abused, this is not a case of moral equivalence. Our task as clinicians and scientists is to whistle blow, and call for honest assessment and reporting from both individuals and organisations worldwide.

Professional organisations may have been guilty of another of Freyd's terms – Institutional Betrayal. They have effectively uncritically endorsed the

FMS line for decades, to the detriment of the abused. It is time for those professional organisations to demonstrate Institutional Courage (see Freyd, 2018), acknowledge their errors, seek the truth and move forward in helping the genuine victims.

In 2018 the British Psychological Society (BPS) was sent a letter from a number of eminent individuals and organisations questioning the wisdom of awarding honours to psychologists who had endorsed scientifically inaccurate statements in promoting a false memory narrative. It took the BPS seven months to reply, stating that the awards were granted for contributions to theoretical work and that "contributions to other organisations, work as an expert witness or otherwise, were not part of the considerations" and that they were "unable to comment on the concerns that you raise ... relating to unscientific claims *and the consequences of those claims*". Well, maybe it is time for the British Psychological Society, the Royal College of Psychiatry, the psychotherapy organisations and all professional organisations internationally to demonstrate Institutional Courage. They need to recognise the appallingly damaging consequences of giving credibility and respectability to individuals and organisations, propagating damaging unscientific views which are categorically contradicted by the actual evidence.

We hope that this book will be a positive force in prompting conscious thought, and attention to the real science and the reality of the scale of CSA and the harm that it does.

So, stories and personal histories are of great importance and value in understanding the mechanisms that allow abuse to take place and in understanding the consequences that can endure over a lifetime. We begin with the remarkable story of Ross Cheit, in discussion with Ashley Conway. He discusses how he came to recall his own abuse, and subsequently demonstrate the reality and accuracy of his recall, and his journey with the topic of recovered memory since that time. In the second chapter Marjorie Orr gives us a startling account of the personal history backgrounds of some of the figures influential in forming the false memory groups. Lynn Crook goes on to explore how accused parents have reframed allegations of abuse as "false memories" using the popular press and other media. Ruth Blizard follows in conversation with Valerie Sinason and describes how the false memory narrative, based on questionable science, came to be used in law courts and elsewhere to discredit the testimony of abuse victims. Winja Buss's chapter is next with an evaluation of false memory research, noticing how easy it is to mislead with evidence inappropriately drawn from laboratory studies (known as a transduction error). In the following chapter Ashley Conway reviews his original work from the 1998 book. His primary conclusion is that he was mistaken and naive in originally thinking that the dispute about traumatic memory had been about science and evidence, rather than a need to deny the accounts of victims. Susie Orbach's chapter on the false memory syndrome is the same as in the original book because we consider it no less relevant today. She examines the part that feminism has played in understanding the extent of abuse against women and children. Ann

Scott adds to her chapter from the first book on the role of language and speech in the false memory debate. She signposts us to some of the more positive changes that have occurred in the last 25 years, particularly the Truth Project as part of the Independent Inquiry into Child Sexual Abuse (in press) in the UK and the #MeToo and Time's Up movements. Brett Kahr gives us an interesting historical perspective on Freud's use of the term repression and concludes that it is possible for repressed events to return to consciousness after long periods of time. Phil Mollon goes on to explore the concept of repression in a clinical setting, both from the patient's perspective and from the clinician hearing their account. Mary Sue Moore discusses the complex functions of memory, and concludes that context is all-important in understanding the polarisation that has occurred in the memory debate. Jennifer Johns's chapter continues Phil Mollon's description of the difficulty for the therapist in hearing the story of abuse. She goes on to describe the terrible countertransference impact that can occur to a therapist, raising the complex issue of difficulty in tolerating uncertainty in knowing what's true. In his chapter Michael Salter examines the meaning of abuse, and the importance of being able to tell one's story. He explores confusion with neoliberalism and the effects of the false memory narrative. Finally, Khadija Rouf and Danny Taggart provide us with a crucial double perspective. Writing as both psychologists and survivors themselves, they explore how we can learn by listening to survivors' accounts, and propose a trauma-informed code of ethics for those working with victims of child sexual abuse.

Our views in this introduction are our personal ones and may not be shared by other contributors to this book. And conversely, whilst the views of all chapter writers are their own, and as co-editors we might not share all the views represented in the book, we can say that everyone writing here shares a concern about the extent of untreated trauma to children and adults in our society. Everyone here is a pioneer who managed to face the reality of trauma and memory.

The painful dynamics of the subject of abuse are played out at every level of society, including the media, academia, consulting rooms, lecture theatres, professional organisations and law courts. There is a danger in professionals forgetting the causes and processes of flights from science and truth.

At the time of writing, the world is feeling threatened by the pandemic of COVID-19. Kucharski (2020) compares the modelling of disease contagion with the spread of viral ideas.

Discussing pandemics, he states

> We get flu epidemics each winter because the virus evolves, making current vaccines less effective … Pandemic preparedness requires a long-term engagement with politically complex, multidimensional problems … In outbreak analysis, the most significant moments aren't the ones where we are right. It's the moments when we realise that we have been wrong … these are the moments we need to reach as early as possible … The moments that let us look back, to work out how outbreaks really

happened in the past. Then look forward, to change how they happen in the future.

Let us look back at our mistakes in our field, and learn. This opportunity now is greater than it has ever been before. When new viral distortions of the science of trauma and memory evolve, let us be prepared – with science and compassion and truth.

Only when blindness is gone can healing truly begin (Freyd & Birrell, 2013).

Whether expressed by apparently well-functioning adults, children, those with learning disabilities, complex PTSD, chronic dissociative states or other mental health problems, our hope is that personal histories will be listened to with the courtesy and respect they need and deserve.

References

Freyd, J. J. (1997). Violations of power, adaptive blindness, and betrayal trauma theory. *Feminism & Psychology*, 7, 22–32.

Freyd, J. J. (2018). When sexual assault victims speak out, their institutions often betray them, *The Conversation*, 11 January 2018. https://theconversation.com/when-sexual-assault-victims-speak-out-their-institutions-often-betray-them-87050

Freyd, J. & Birrell, P. (2013). *Blind to Betrayal*. London: John Wiley & Sons.

Independent Inquiry Child Sexual Abuse (IICSA). (In progress at the time of going to press). iicsa.org.uk.

Kucharski, A. (2020). *The Rules of Contagion*. London: Profile Books.

Loftus, E. & Pickrell, J. (1995). The formation of false memories. *Psychiatric Annals*, 25, 720–725. http://users.ecs.soton.ac.uk/harnad/Papers/Py104/loftus.mem.html

Office of National Statistics (2020). Child Abuse Extent and Nature, England and Wales: Year Ending March 2019. London: ONS.

Reinders, A. A. T. S., Willemsen, A. T. M., Vos, H. P. J., den Boer, J. A. & Nijenhuis, E. R. S. (2012). Fact or Factitious? A Psychobiological Study of Authentic and Simulated Dissociative Identity States. *PLoS ONE*, 7(6): e39279. https://doi.org/10.1371/journal.pone.0039279

Sinason, V. (Ed.) (1998). *Memory in Dispute*. London: Karnac.

Chapter 1

In conversation with Ross Cheit

Ashley Conway

In this chapter, Ross is in discussion with Ashley Conway. He describes his personal journey with recovered memory, and the reaction to it. He relates the difficulty in providing enough evidence to make the false memory advocates acknowledge the veracity of survivors' accounts. He also discusses false memory syndrome supporters' success in the media and the difficulty in responding because of libel law.

ASHLEY: First, I know that you are not a psychologist – what are your professional qualifications?

ROSS: I have a PhD in Public Policy and I have a law degree. I am professor of Political Science and International & Public Affairs at Brown University, Rhode Island, USA.

ASHLEY: What led you to write your brilliant book, *The Witch Hunt Narrative* (Cheit, 2014a)? Where is the beginning of this story?

ROSS: It began with personal experience and I have made no secret of that fact. But when I look back to 1992, I was initially mortified at the thought people would know about this and not believe me. Anyway, I woke up one day with a strong recollection from a dream about a man I had not thought of for 20 years and I felt sick to my stomach. I thought of this man who was a counsellor at a summer camp I went to and realised he had sexually abused me. Had someone asked me directly before this if I had ever been sexually abused as a kid I would have said no. So, I woke up with this sick feeling, felt mortified and then my curiosity took over. I wanted to know what had happened and where he was, and my questions made me want to investigate this. There were times I felt I had prepared all my life for this moment as I had mustered skills that could help with this. I had practised law in Berkeley, California, where I had worked with a good private investigator and I had him find former boys, now men, who had been at the San Francisco Boys Chorus summer camp. He did a brilliant job of tracking down people who had been in this camp in the 1960s and I contacted people out of the blue asking if they remembered me. I then asked if they remembered Bill Farmer and I quickly discovered other victims of Bill Farmer, including a counsellor

DOI: 10.4324/9781003193159-2

who had told the director of the camp. I ultimately proved a wide amount of abuse and cover-up. It happened to be that the final year of the camp was 1968, when I had just turned 13.

ASHLEY: You found other people who had that experience?

ROSS: And other counsellors who did it. The private investigator tracked Bill Farmer's history and he had gone from town to town where he held himself out as a religious figure, and he had been run out of various towns where he had been found out. There was a place where a judge's son was abused, and the judge ordered him out. He did this five or six times. I will try and wrap this up, as this story could take the whole hour of our interview. It is compelling and involved issues after he was apprehended that were remarkable. Anyway, we found out where he was in a small town in Oregon and I had a phone number. I called that number as I wanted to confront him. And one night I got an answer. His wife answered. I said to tell him it is someone who knows him from a long time ago. He says "hello" and I say "hello, this is Ross Cheit. Do you remember me?" And he replies, "Yes. Yes. But I picture you as a 12-year-old", which turned my stomach. I confronted him in direct terms and he asked if he could call me back and I said no this was his only chance to speak to me. My father, my late father, not an emotive man, said that this was the most remarkable conversation he ever heard. I didn't know if taping the call was legal but it turns out I was in a state where there was one-party consent for recording. He fully confessed what he did to me and other kids. He then disappeared from that address and that state, so it was hard to trace him, but we did eventually find him in Corpus Christi. I went to the Chorus with an incredible amount of information. I had information about other victims, and I had statements from counsellors and I had a tape-recorded confession. What did I get in response? The lawyer for the Chorus said that the organisation had done "so well for so many kids", and they criticised me for wanting to damage their reputation. The idea they just wanted to get rid of me was stunning, so we had a lawsuit. That would have been 1994. Right after we filed the suit, they went to a friendly judge and asked for the files to be sealed, claiming it would damage their reputation if it was made public. And the judge agreed without us there. I had so many things going for me, including a brother who is a clever lawyer and former journalist. We arranged to appeal the seal and we knew that all of the papers would be public at the appellate level for at least a day. So we made sure that a journalist saw the documents the day they were public. Within a year the Chorus settled with me, as I wanted an apology. In my mind it was never about money. It was about acknowledgement. But they still honour the woman who covered this up, so I was not as successful as I wanted. But I succeeded in many ways.

ASHLEY: And what happened to Bill Farmer?

ROSS: We found him in Texas and served him with papers in my civil lawsuit. He never made an appearance, and I received what is known as a default judgement. I still had to appear and testify, and the judge awarded around $450,000. I never collected a cent.

California changed its statute of limitations during that time, as well, allowing for criminal charges in recovered memory cases to go forward if corroborated by multiple sources. I got two other men to stand with me and convinced a District Attorney to file criminal charges. Farmer was arrested in Texas and fought extradition, spending 17 days, I think, in a Texas jail. He was sent to California and immediately released because the lower court judge ruled that it was not clear whether the legislature really meant for the law to be retroactive.

Years later one of his kids rang me up to get help to have a restraining order so he couldn't visit his grandchildren, and another kid rang me years later not wanting their dad to be on a transplant list. Since the lawsuit, I volunteered for years at the prison working with sex offenders as I wanted to understand how this man could do such things. And that work also gave me some empathy. Child molesters are responsible for what they do and should be punished, but they do not start out choosing this as a way of life. Many have had a horrid start in life themselves. But I don't want to carry on about Bill Farmer.

ASHLEY: Yes. We could carry on for the whole conversation just on that …

On the topic of public disclosure by victims of abuse, it has been so powerful to watch the victims in the recent Nassar sentencing hearing make their statements [Larry Nassar was an American gymnastics national team doctor. He was accused of assaulting at least 200 young women and girls. He admitted to some of the accusations, for which he has received lengthy prison sentences]. I hope that will help a shift of views here in the UK. People having the courage to tell their stories, as you did.

ROSS: I was just compelled to do what I did. I never called it courage. When I went to a lawyer the first thing he said to me was that I would be believed as I was a man. I knew intellectually that women were discounted but that hit me hard. I was so worried I would not be believed. But then thinking I was a white male with tenure and resources so if I did not do this, who would? I paid a real price in some ways, but it was also very successful.

ASHLEY: I have great respect for that Ross. I occasionally have colleagues asking me why I have done this work for 20 years. I suppose I have wanted to understand why people who disclose abuse have been called fantasists, or are accused of having "false memories". My colleagues ask me why I want to be involved in such a contentious and demanding field.

ROSS: I had a senior colleague who asked, "are you still studying that?" with disdain. He could not put words to it.

ASHLEY: In the coverage of that hearing I heard a definition of being complicit: Knowing what is going on, and doing nothing. I give the question back – and ask: How can you be a psychologist, understanding the reality of dissociative amnesia and recall, and not say anything? Why do we let people believe this does not happen, and why do we allow those who deny and minimise to have such a loud voice? I don't understand that as a professional.

I remember reading a comment about you, from a FMS (false memory syndrome) advocate, I think, implying that your account was not accurate. What do you say to that?

ROSS: The FMS has not denied that I was abused. But they have tried to discount my academic work because of my personal experience. They have also said "you must have remembered all along and were pretending you didn't", although there was no legal advantage for doing that and no reason I would have delayed taking the actions that I did when I remembered. One other critic, Mark Pendergrast (a freelance writer – see, e.g. Pendergrast, 2017), has said, "What happened wasn't traumatic, and it only happened once" and therefore it was just "regular forgetting". I have no idea how he can claim it only happened once. Anyway, they can't deny the reality. But they have said that I never proved I forgot! How can you prove you forgot? I say, "look what I did when I remembered!"

ASHLEY: Bessel Van der Kolk (2015) makes a straight-forward point, that when we talk about traumatic amnesia in soldiers who have been in combat no one seems to argue with that. Early on in my professional life I worked with banks and other organisations where there had been armed robberies. I talked to many, many victims, and learned how they often had memory blanks and struggled to remember detail. They might have remembered seeing the gun, but not how many robbers there were.

ROSS: They do attack the reality of this. Elaine Showalter has claimed that PTSD in the context of military people is phoney. There really are deniers of all of this. Already one of the Nassar victims has been accused of "illusory" memory. Mark Pendergrast said when one victim used the word "suppressed" that her memory must be "illusory". No one in their right mind felt any of those victims were not genuine. This claim is so preposterous – I want this largely publicised.

ASHLEY: I guess that you are familiar with the Nicole Taus case? [Nicole Taus was the subject of a case study, who was assured anonymity. Elizabeth Loftus published information which made her identity very much easier to discover. See Kluemper, (2014). Taus now holds three postgraduate degrees in psychology].

ROSS: I wrote why this was unethical from a journalistic point of view (Cheit, 2014b).

ASHLEY: I sent you a tiny analysis of Elizabeth Loftus's TED lecture (Loftus, 2013) where, in my opinion, she inexcusably put Taus's name up on a slide.

ROSS: I was on a panel with Nicole Taus last year and she is now talking out publicly. However, they destroyed her life in many ways. In that TED talk Elizabeth Loftus makes statements about the facts of the case that are simply untrue. She said the mother was accused based on a recovered memory, rather than the statements of a little girl when she was 6 years old.

ASHLEY: I Have heard of Nicole Taus's case being referred to as a "black swan case". You are another black swan aren't you?

ROSS: Yes. I would rather be called that than a poster boy! [Both men laugh]

ASHLEY: There seem to be a lot of black swans! I wonder if you have a way of making sense of this? For example, for some of those "experts" who so vehemently deny the existence of recovered memory, do you think that there could be any amount of evidence that could cause them to say, "Ah, this person has recovered a genuine, accurate memory, and they were abused?"

ROSS: I think that is the litmus test for if someone is in any way open-minded. There are FMS proponents who allow that there might be a case that is true, but Loftus and Pendergrast are in the position where nothing will persuade them. I can't locate where Loftus said it but she asked somewhere, "where are the corroborated cases if this is true?" and eventually I told her there were 100 on my website, but it could not persuade her.

ASHLEY: So, for me a big question is this: Is this about science? We are doing this interview for a book that I think is extraordinary. It started out being a second edition of a book written 20 years ago, and I felt rather than rewrite I wanted to review my old chapter. And my conclusion, sadly, is that this denial continues and I was naive. I thought it was about evidence and science. Now I realise it isn't.

ROSS: I study politics and in some ways this is about politics and not science, although there are scientists in this area. The most discouraging issue is that some of these scientists, like Ceci and Bruck and Loftus, are people with high prestige scientific jobs who are not acting like scientists in this area. I have colleagues who admire Loftus for her good scientific work on the fallibility of evidence, but in this area she is an advocate.

ASHLEY: Personally, I don't think laboratory research involving implanting memories has much to inform us about traumatic experience and memory of trauma.

ROSS: Gail Goodman understands children and abuse and has done some good laboratory experiments that get at this. [Gail Goodman is Distinguished Professor of Psychology at the University of California. See, e.g. Howe, Goodman, & Cicchetti, 2008]. She has been mercilessly attacked and they went after her in a way that scared other people from doing that research.

ASHLEY: And Maggie Bruck (see, e.g. Ceci & Brook, 1995) … you mentioned her recently. I realise that her work is more about implanting a story than recovered memory, but there are similar themes – what would it take to consider a different interpretation (e.g. the account is true)?

ROSS: Yes, her work constitutes what I would call "credibility discounting" of children. Her laboratory work seems devoted to "proving" that children are highly suggestible. And she testifies to that effect for defendants which is, of course, something quite different from doing experiments. My research focuses on the kinds of cases in which she appears, so I take your question as "In what kind of case would she ever find a child's word credible?" The answer seems to be that she is always against the child, no matter what. I found a case where she impugned the child's testimony even though there was an adult witness to the abuse. I also found that she misrepresented the underlying facts in the Kelly Michaels case in order to get colleagues to sign the famous "Concerned Scientists" brief that was filed with the court. Her book with Ceci (Ceci & Bruck, 1995) included excerpts from interviews in that case that were doctored; it took years of work to get to those transcripts and make this discovery.

I felt I could not publish my book without giving her a chance to respond to what I found. So I sat in her office in Baltimore and I formed my questions very carefully. Eventually, I handed her a copy from the actual transcript and the part in her book and asked why they did not match. She asked, "How did you get this?" The transcript had been sealed and I explained that I had reached an agreement with the state that provided me with access to the transcripts subject to a promise, contained in the Human Subjects Protocol approved at my university, not to reveal any of the children's names. Her response to that information was to say, "That's rotten". I guess she thought it was rotten that someone was able to check her work. She promised to get back to me with an explanation, but that was one of many things she promised to follow-up on, and never did.

ASHLEY: Isn't that a marvellous way that someone from a discipline outside of psychology can use their skills to throw light on something that would otherwise have been in darkness forever?

ROSS: There is no question that it was possible for me to do this work because I am not in the field. There are many academic psychologists who are aware of the ways in which Elizabeth Loftus has acted unethically and unscientifically, but they don't dare speak out. They don't want to be blackballed, have papers rejected, etc. I didn't have any of those things at stake. They can't affect my academic life, but if I was in psychology they could. I found a letter that Maggie Bruck wrote to the editors of peer-reviewed journals saying Gail Goodman was an extremist "who always thinks the children are telling the truth". That is demonstrably not true; Goodman is a highly credible researcher who just happens to disagree with Bruck. I can see why psychologists keep their mouths shut.

ASHLEY: I am really interested in that, and I don't know if it is the same in the USA. Here the FMS zealots represent only a small proportion of psychologists, but have a loud and powerful voice. For some reason Elizabeth Loftus has a place on the editorial board of our house journal, The Psychologist, and one of the British False Memory Society (BFMS) advisers was given a very important role on a British Psychological Society committee. I wrote him a reasonably polite letter, pointing out that there were factually wrong statements on the BFMS site, and I thought it ethically important that he ensures the accuracy of statements made as facts. I got a letter back saying I was being a bully and he did not want to hear from me again.

ROSS: Wow.

ASHLEY: And our professional society, the British Psychological Society is affected. Their position is very unclear. They seem to give a voice to those who deny the reality of traumatic amnesia, while offering little guidance to victims of abuse or those trying to help them.

A few years ago, here in the UK a woman committed suicide mid-trial of her abuser. Her suicide was kept from the jury until after the trial. Her abuser was found guilty, and it turned out that she was advised not to have any therapy, as it might have disadvantaged the prosecution of the case. That narrative, that if you have therapy the defence can use that fact to discredit the account, is so toxic.

ROSS: Before Larry Nassar, it was Jerry Sandusky, and Mark Pendergrast's (2017) book argues he is innocent, as some of those boys went to therapists.

ASHLEY: I find myself reacting to that emotionally. I find it very hard to know what to say to that.

ROSS: It is awful and stunning. Elizabeth Loftus, who offered that claim in the Sandusky case, has been less successful in court than in the media. The judge in the Sandusky case said that her theory was based "on an uncritical review of an absurdly incomplete record carefully dissected to include only pieces of information". He rejected it entirely. I know many cases where she has lost and she never talks about those.

ASHLEY: How do these people still have such a loud voice? In the London Evening Standard a journalist wrote of the Weinstein case: "I suspect that false memory syndrome has increased the velocity of these tales ..." I thought – the FMS zealots have got their story so deeply embedded into social consciousness, that a journalist with no knowledge puts that into the middle of an article. It is a brilliant PR job. They are so good at it.

ROSS: No question. They have been very successful with the media and the media loves an innocence story. "Convicted man is guilty as charged" is not a story. But someone claiming to be falsely accused and convicted is loved and there are structural reasons why that story gets told so often. The defence in America can speak to the press but the prosecutor is prohibited by ethics. Defence people are out there pushing a slanted version of the facts and even more so after convictions because prosecutors have won and don't speak. But the defence twists things more and more so that by the time 20 years have gone the twists are outrageous but there is no one to correct the record unless someone like me comes along.

ASHLEY: Can I ask you about the Eileen Franklin case? [In 1990, based upon the recovered memories of Eileen Franklin, her father, George Franklin was found guilty of the murder of 8-year-old Susan Nason. The conviction was overturned in 1995].

ROSS: Of course. I have got to write about this, as he has been called "exoner-ated". One of the two reasons his conviction was overturned was because of his own self-incrimination. The Appeals court said that should not have been allowed in. He incriminated himself and the idea that someone can be exonerated when they incriminated themselves … A Michigan law school professor has created a list of "exonerations". But of course, you can have a conviction overturned when you are still guilty.

ASHLEY: To sum that up – in a case where an issue of the legal process has meant someone is free to go, that then becomes described as exoneration?

ROSS: Those kinds of constitutional structures prefer ten guilty to be free rather than one innocent convicted. I agree with that, but when the guilty go free we should not call them innocent. It is very hard to write about the guilty who go free because of the libel law. If you say the conviction was overturned but there was evidence of guilt you can say that, but not "they are guilty".

ASHLEY: In both the UK and USA the false memory societies were founded by people accused of child sexual abuse.

ROSS: Absolutely.

ASHLEY: And they are there to represent the interests of people accused of sexual abuse. It needs to be acknowledged. Even 20 years ago I realised it was easy for the press to report that someone is falsely accused, whereas the abused and therapist get no voice.

ROSS: There are a variety of structural reasons why that story gets told more often, and that is one of them. If you went to a newspaper and said, "my father abused me and never got arrested", they won't publish it.

ASHLEY: Do you have any solution to that?

ROSS: I don't. But I think the problem begins with the media. The *LA Times* got a Pulitzer for attacking their own coverage of the McMartin Preschool case. Their media critic wrote that in the first six months of that case no journalist lit a match within a mile of the prosecutor's feet. I think he was right about that. The press repeated everything with full incredulity. But by the end of the same case, things had reversed. Now journalists don't light a match within a mile of the defence lawyer's feet. We have gone from one end to another and I am waiting for it to swing back.

ASHLEY: Do you think it will move back?

ROSS: I guess I do. I think it is moving right now. But I am attentive to people like Pendergrast who is already impugning a Nassar victim. But this moment is different.

ASHLEY: In your case – no one has said it never happened to you? But rather that there is something wrong with your memory? Is that right?

ROSS: Yes – they say I remembered it all along and am lying or it was just ordinary forgetting. To me this is the Catch-22 people. Richard McNally, a Harvard psychologist, features a PowerPoint slide that says, "Trauma is memorable". Okay, but how can you say that when someone forgets trauma it is just "regular forgetting"? That is their claim about every documented case of recovered memory.

ASHLEY: Does it offend you? This implication you are lying.

ROSS: Sure. The implication is made that a civil lawsuit would not have been possible had I remembered all along. But that ignores the concept of comprehension-based statutes of limitation. And my suit was never about money anyway! I got a 500,000-dollar judgement against him, but I never got a penny as he didn't have money. I knew that; I wanted acknowledgement and accountability.

ASHLEY: Your account reminds me of what I hear about Nicole Taus. That this is not about money.

ROSS: Taus filed an ethics complaint, and got the wrath of Elizabeth Loftus in return. It should be noted that the University of Washington told Loftus she needed ethics training. Loftus left the university in protest. Taus's civil suit was a last resort to gain some sense of justice.

ASHLEY: Anything more you want to say?

ROSS: I do want to say – and I think this is important – the idea that a person might go to a therapist and come out with a false belief about something is possible. It is not impossible. I grant, as they will not in the instance of recovered memory, that there are cases that fit that description. I don't think there were ever thousands of them but the idea that a vulnerable person with a single-minded therapist could lead to a toxic result is true; that is also true in other areas of therapy that have nothing to do with memory. It is important to say that. There can be members of the FMSF who come from a righteous place of injustice. The problem is there is no question but that the organisation also provides cover for the guilty, it attracts the guilty and they welcome all comers without question. That is really a problem.

ASHLEY: I absolutely agree with that. That kind of reasonableness. Why does it have to be polarised? Why can't it be acknowledged that both false and recovered memory can be real? That memory can be malleable in different directions?

ROSS: The world is complicated.

ASHLEY: People who are traumatised can be amnesic to parts or the whole of the event. And they might recall it later. Why is that so hard to acknowledge?

ROSS: Why can't the press understand the Goldwater Rule, which has been discussed recently because of Trump; it evolved from psychiatrists commenting on Barry Goldwater's mental health when he was running for president. It was felt you can't make public statements about people you don't know and have not analysed. But the FMSF seems to think you can diagnose someone you have never met.

ASHLEY: That is a brilliant place to end.

ROSS: It is stunning when you take it apart, and realise that people have not understood.

ASHLEY: Thank you I really appreciate it.

ROSS: And I would love to connect in the UK in the next few years. In some ways my life is too isolated.

ASHLEY: Ross, thank you very much.

References

Ceci, S. & Bruck, M. (1995). *Jeopardy in the Courtroom: A Scientific Analysis of Children's Testimony.* Washington, DC: American Psychological Association.

Cheit, R. (2014a). *The Witch-Hunt Narrative: Politics, Psychology and the Sexual Abuse of Children.* Oxford: Oxford University Press.

Cheit, R. (2014b). Research Ethics and Case Studies in Psychology: A Commentary on *Taus v. Loftus. Journal of Interpersonal Violence,* 29, 3290–3307.

Howe, M. L., Goodman, G. S. & Cicchetti, D. (Eds.). (2008). *Stress, Trauma, and Children's Memory Development: Neurobiological, Cognitive, Clinical and Legal Perspectives.* New York: Oxford University Press.

Kluemper, N. S. (2014). One woman's account of having her confidentiality violated. *Journal of Interpersonal Violence,* 29, 3232–3244

Loftus, E. (2013). *How Reliable is your Memory?* TED Global talk, June 2013. https://www.ted.com/talks/elizabeth_loftus_the_fiction_of_memory

Pendergrast, M. (2017). *The Most Hated Man in America: Jerry Sandusky and the Rush to Judgement.* Mechanicsburg: Sunbury Press.

Van Der Kolk, B. (2015). *The Body Keeps the Score: Brain, Mind, and Body in the Healing of Trauma.* London: Penguin.

Chapter 2

False memory syndrome movement

The origins and the promoters

Marjorie Orr

Marjorie Orr updates her chapter from Memory in Dispute. In presenting a history of the false memory syndrome Movements, she looks closely at their origins and promoters. She provides comments from the adult children of the False Memory Syndrome Foundation member parents as well as the media involvement and response and the failure of false memory syndrome scientific arguments.

The man credited with coining the term "false memory syndrome" was the late Dr Ralph Underwager, a minister and psychologist, who since the 1970s had been a defence witness for those accused of child sexual abuse. He was one of the creators of the False Memory Syndrome Foundation (FMSF) in 1992 along with Peter Freyd, an academic mathematician facing allegations of sexual abuse by a daughter; with his wife Pamela Freyd also taking a leading role. Their fledgeling society attracted other parents accused of child sexual abuse and prompted similar set-ups in the UK and other countries. In order to bolster their credibility, advisory boards were put in place filled with eminent academics and psychology professionals.

Pulitzer-prize-winning journalist Mike Stanton wrote in 1997:

> Rarely has such a strange and little-understood organisation had such a profound effect on media coverage of such a controversial matter. Most reporters don't realise the FMSF's impressive array of scientific advisers represent just one part of a broad spectrum of psychological thought. The board is dominated by research psychologists and biologically oriented therapists – inclined to seek physical reasons for problems and to treat them with drugs.
>
> (Stanton, 1997)

A similar conclusion was expressed by UK media scholar Professor Jenny Kitzinger: "How was a small and unofficial organisation able to achieve such remarkable success in defining a new social problem and attracting media attention?" (Kitzinger, 1998).

Accuracy About Abuse was set up in 1994 as an information service with the aim of counteracting the misuse of "false memory" as a wholesale defence

DOI: 10.4324/9781003193159-3

against allegations of sexual abuse, even where those alleging childhood abuse had never forgotten, or been in therapy. It also publicised the beliefs of many of those espousing the "false memory" cause.

In 1990 and 1992 Ralph Underwager and his wife Hollida Wakefield co-authored articles with Benjamin Rossen, a board member of *Paidika*, a self-styled journal of paedophilia; and they subsequently gave an explicit interview to *Paidika* saying that paedophilia could be seen as a responsible choice; that having sex with children could be seen as "part of God's will"; and that feminists were jealous of men's ability to bond with boys. Underwager later said he was not misquoted by the magazine. He was forced to resign, although his wife continued on the FMSF Advisory Board (Geraci, 1993). Their interview was reprinted in full in *Dares to Speak*, a 1997 book by Joseph Geraci, editor of *Paidika* (Geraci, 1997).

To be noted, Underwager had previously given oral and written evidence to the 1987 UK Cleveland Inquiry and was described by the chairperson, Lord Justice Butler-Sloss, as a "valuable and important witness". In his oral evidence he asserted the following as proven by research – abused children are not secretive: cannot feel shame or embarrassment before the age of 9 or 11; the recidivism rate for abusers is 1% to 2%; abused children are rarely threatened; 5% of claims of abuse are probably well-founded as judged by the conviction rate; and there is no therapeutic benefit in an abused child expressing their feelings afterwards to a psychiatrist.

In April of 1994 American Appeal Court judges threw out Underwager's defamation suit against Anna Salter, a child psychologist, who had written a highly critical expose of his scholarship and methods. The three judges said that Anna Salter was not malicious in concluding that Underwager was "a hired gun who makes a living by deceiving judges about the state of medical knowledge and thus assisting child molesters to evade punishment". They were clear that the law would not challenge her in continuing to say so. In 1993 a Canadian Court similarly found Underwager's testimony "replete with misinterpretation, misquoting and reliance upon information that is not empirical data" (Salter, 1991; Underwager and Wakefield v. Salter et al., 1993).

The other co-founders of the FMS Foundation in Philadelphia, Pamela and Peter Freyd, describe themselves as innocents much-maligned, and founded the False Memory Syndrome Foundation after an allegation of sexual abuse was made privately against Peter Freyd by one of their two adult daughters, Jennifer. In 1991 Pamela Freyd published a thinly disguised and highly biased account of her position under the name of Jane Doe, which she widely disseminated in 1991 and 1992 to many, including her daughter's colleagues.

The American media gave her parents almost unquestioning support until their daughter, Professor Jennifer Freyd, a tenured professor and cognitive psychology expert in her 30s, reluctantly felt obliged to speak up publicly to stop the damage she felt her parents and their organisation were doing to abuse victims (Freyd, 1993).

She spoke not of the core "recovered" abuse memories themselves which she rightly felt to be private, but the parts of childhood she clearly remembered in which she had felt sexual boundaries were constantly crossed; in which she felt invaded, controlled, intimidated and manipulated.

In her one public lecture she told a family story in which her parents grew up as step-brother and step-sister from a young age. The grandparents had an affair which culminated after 11 years in marriage, at which time Pamela and Peter Freyd also married aged 18 and 20. Professor Freyd recollected her father speaking openly of his own childhood homosexual liaison as an 11-year-old with a paedophile artist. She remembered being made to dance nude in front of him aged 9 with a friend; of being taught to kiss on the mouth "like an adult" for a school play aged 11 in front of the cast. She made particular mention of a mould of his penis and testicles, which she saw on one occasion on the mantelpiece in the sitting room. She says he continually made sexual comments which were regarded as normal in the family, for example, that the family dog could sense her sister's sexual interest in men, and he explained in front of his 2-year-old grandson that turkey basters were used by lesbians to inseminate themselves. He drank heavily through her childhood and was hospitalised for alcoholism.

Jennifer Freyd, though highly motivated as a student did struggle with some aspects of her life. She has described her mother's invasion of her privacy as horrifying, horribly invasive and violating. She has said that she chose to speak about these matters "because I hope what I have to share will help ... other abused children and adult survivors of abuse" (Freyd & Birrell, 2013). Both Pamela and Peter Freyd now deny the family was dysfunctional. The other sister and Peter Freyd's brother (his only sibling) both support Jennifer Freyd. None of them are in direct contact with the parents.

Peter Freyd's brother, William, wrote an open letter to a TV station after a slanted documentary on recovered memories. He wrote:

> There is no doubt in my mind that there was severe abuse in the home of Peter and Pam, while they were raising their daughters ... The False Memory Syndrome Foundation is a fraud designed to deny a reality that Peter and Pam have spent most of their lives trying to escape ... That the False Memory Syndrome Foundation has been able to excite so much media attention has been a great surprise to those of us who would like to admire and respect the objectivity of people in the media. Neither Peter's mother (who was also mine), nor his daughters, nor I have wanted anything to do with Peter and Pam for periods of time ranging up to more than two decades. We do not understand why you would "buy" such a flawed story.
>
> (Freyd, 1995)

Jennifer Freyd also emphasised in her lecture that she did not recover her memories under hypnosis. She went to a mainstream clinical psychologist in a medical practice and the memories started to emerge after the first session. Yet she said:

> apparently my mother has suggested to many people that my memories were the result of therapeutic intervention, even hypnosis. This makes me wonder about the claims of other parents associated with FMSF ... It is as if the weight of a whole Foundation (false memory syndrome) stands behind my mother's frenzied denial of my reality.

Fourteen months after the original private accusation of abuse Pamela Freyd incorporated the False Memory Syndrome Foundation; and later said of Ralph Underwager and his wife Hollida Wakefield, "there are not enough words to thank (them) ... for the loving professional support that they have given to the FMS Foundation to help us become an independent organisation. We would not exist without them".

Professor Jennifer Freyd has spent three decades researching and writing extensively on sexual abuse and memory. Some of this work predates the formation of the FMSF, and was perhaps one of the triggers for its launch. In her 1996 book *Betrayal Trauma: The Logic of Forgetting Childhood Abuse.* she argues that

> under certain conditions, such as abuse by a close caregiver, amnesia for the abuse is an adaptive response, for amnesia may allow a dependent child to remain attached to – and thus elicit at least some degree of life-sustaining nurturing and protection from – his or her abusive caregiver.
>
> (Freyd, 1996)

The *New York Times* book review described the book as a

> thoughtful, judicious and thorough scholarly analysis of a subject that has generated more heat than light ... her work serves as a salutary reminder that if treated as serious science rather than media hoopla, the recovered memory debate could provide a significant window on mind-brain relationships ...
>
> (Bickerton, 1997)

In the UK, the British False Memory Society (BFMS) was set up by Roger Scotford, an ex-naval engineer, who publicly admitted that he was accused by two of his three daughters of abusing them. In various press interviews initially under different pseudonyms – "Tony", "James", "Bill" – he says that he had a happy and involved relationship with the family throughout childhood and beyond. Only when his middle daughter went to a homoeopath for an unrelated problem did any thought of abuse arise. From this he concluded that she was brainwashed by the therapist. He vehemently denied any abuse took place.

Both daughters insisted they were significantly unhappy throughout childhood. Recurring descriptions are of being lonely, numb, cut off, depressed, and on occasions wanting to die. One described herself as "the one who did not exist".

The middle daughter did go to a mainstream analyst in her late teens for about six months. On relating a sexual dream about her father, she was told that this was a perfectly normal fantasy for girls to have. When she was 27 she agreed to accompany her father on a brief holiday to understand why she disliked him and to resolve their differences. During a tense few days, she was conscious of her body beginning to react strangely.

In the following week she had an appointment with a homoeopath for the thrush which had, along with kidney and urethral infections, been a recurring problem for most of her life. When she arrived very agitated by her holiday experience she was greeted, she said, by the first person in her life who really wanted to listen to her. "It was completely unprompted what I came up with", she said. As with Jennifer Freyd, there was no hypnotherapy. That was the start of a long difficult process of recovering what she believed to be memories of abuse. Neither she nor her sister withdrew their stories over the 25 years following.

After Accuracy About Abuse was formed in 1994, many adult children whose parents were members of the British False Memory Society made contact, scared and outraged by their parents' one-sided stories appearing unquestioned on TV and in press features.

The statements below were volunteered by adult children who were for the most part frightened of coming out of hiding; some changed their addresses to escape their parents. Few of them wished to be involved in a public slanging match, and the media were, in any event, reluctant to print their side of the story because of the libel risk.

- "I have always remembered though she says it was all the therapist's doing. I confronted her privately but she has gone around broadcasting it, which is very embarrassing for me and humiliating. Luckily my father, who is divorced, has been a tower of strength for me and I am much more confident now".
- "I am extremely angry that my private anguish and grief are being hawked around … My parents have joined the False Memory Society and constantly bombard me with their literature. It seems to me that the counselling community is not standing up for itself against these attacks".
- "I have memories of abuse but my parents are now persecuting me with the FMS claims and I fear that this will now help them destroy any piece of happiness that I manage to build for myself. I am finding that now they have another reason to persecute my life although I have never threatened them with anything. I only ever wanted to talk to them about childhood memories which of course they deny. As a child my father said he would kill me if I told. Now he says he will destroy me unless I come back into the family and deny".
- "I never had hypnotherapy and had not really totally forgotten. I have been threatened over the past 2 years with being sued for defamation if I

speak out. He even suggested that since I had confronted him and he had a heart condition, it was really attempted murder. I have heard recently from my ex-therapist that her organisation was lectured to by a false memory speaker who said they had a blacklist of therapists. This woman who literally saved my life is now very edgy".

- "I was my father's victim before I could walk and he kept sexually abusing me well into my childhood. He threatened me never to speak about it and I had no choice but to suppress my experiences. With the truth hidden I was able to survive in the family facade, which grew into the 'happy' family. I began to let the memories in when I was 21. It was a gradual and frightening process even with the help of psychotherapy. There is no hypnosis. I found out afterwards my story had been on TV. I was horrified. I knew nothing about the programme and had been given no opportunity to tell my story. I felt helpless and silenced".

- "My parents have been very active in the FMS in the UK. I find it deeply upsetting and disturbing. I think there is a real danger that the media and the general public will get "compassion fatigue" and that the issue of abuse will be ignored, trivialised and marginalised again which would be terrible. I also feel powerless for reasons of confidentiality a real fear that if I wrote what happened to me. I would be sued by my family. I do not feel that I am free to speak. When I read through the articles in the press it makes me feel quite anxious and puts me in touch with my parents and their persistent actions to try to make me recant".

- "We have been told that we are included as an FMS 'case', although none of their own criteria for inclusion were met. Our close friends, neighbours and relatives, even my G.P. and employer, are bombarded with FMS literature which has done considerable damage with letters saying I am mentally sick. This means I am having to constantly defend myself against the abuse for which I should have no guilt".

- "My father was physically abusive to all family members. My memories come back before I went into therapy. He was an exhibitionist at home which he said was healthy, and a liar. I used to get hysterical if I couldn't lock the bathroom door. The rest of the family support me".

- A close childhood friend and neighbour: "My parents stopped being friends with her parents because like a lot of others in the neighbourhood they felt uneasy about the atmosphere in the family. There was always something odd. Sex was openly talked about in front of the children in a strange way and the father seemed to be obsessed with her (the daughter's) sex life and the way her body was developing" (Accuracy About Abuse Newsletter, 2 June 1994; AAA10 March 1996).

These quotes are from people who found themselves in the Kafkaesque situation of having confronted their parents privately and then finding their parents' version of their family history being paraded as the truth and accepted, largely unquestioningly, by journalists, the general public and many professionals. I was refused permission to tell their stories, even anonymously, at a UKCP conference in 1995, on "Memories of Abuse: False Memory, Recovered memory and the problems of child abuse". The chairman deemed it unacceptable for me to "attack" the FMS parents.

Membership figures for both the US and British false memory associations were regularly exaggerated in the media. Peter Freyd publicly admitted in 1995 that the paid membership for the American FMSF was around 2500, not 16,000 as was widely thought. Roger Scotford has said that in December 1994 the BFMS had 230 paid members, not 650 as had been quoted. The British Psychological Society Report (Morton et al., 1995), which supported the idea that both repressed memory of sexual abuse and false memory were real occurrences found the BFMS's membership files to be sketchy and inconsistent. In three-quarters of the cases there was not even a mention of memory recovery.

Roger Scotford, the chairman/founder of the UK BFMS, aligned himself to the Children of God cult leaders, Rachel and Gideon Scott, whom he accompanied to two conferences, including one in Utrecht attacking Child Protection, in which Dr Ralph Underwager, Hollida Wakefield, Dr Richard Ofshe were principal speakers. His support provoked the resignation of Dr Elizabeth Tylden, a BFMS advisory board member. She told me:

> I became aware that the FMS were actively supporting 'The Family', formerly Children of God. I have experience of gross sexual impropriety to which children in this organisation have been exposed. Roger Scotford (the chairman) wrote to me after I had resigned saying he was going to support cult members who had been falsely accused.

An *Observer* newspaper survey on cults wrote:

> It is difficult to find a cult with a worse reputation than the Children of God (now known as the Family) – a teenage girl was recently awarded £5000 by the British Criminal Injuries Compensation Board having been abused by members of the sect from the age of three. It is estimated that of the 9000 current members of The Family, 6,000 are children; many of them the off-spring of the sect's "Hookers for Christ" campaign in the 1970s and 1980s in which women members seduced potential converts and bore their chil-dren … Members were urged to "share" each other's wives and husbands, pornography was circulated, sex with children was elliptically condoned and "God's Whores" were instructed to pick up men in discos and bars.
>
> (Observer, 1995)

Two other prominent UK BFMS Advisory Board members Peter Fonagy and Gisli Gudjonsson also resigned, though others remained in place, including two and a BFMS medical consultant who made up half the membership of a volun-teer committee for a UK Royal College of Psychiatrists working party on child sexual abuse in 1996/7, chaired by Professor Sydney Brandon. Accuracy About Abuse was asked to provide the names of abuse survivors with corroborated recovered memories for the interview. Assurances were given that the interviews would be sympathetically carried out by a "neutral" psychiatrist, experienced in the field and that there would be no False Memory Society connection. When it turned out that the sole nominated interviewer, Dr Richard Green, was an advisory board member of the UK BFMS and the USA FMSF, our co-operation was withdrawn. The draft report subsequently written stated that no corroborated memory cases could be found; and was so out of line with clinical experience and recent research evidence that several sections of the Royal College of Psychiatrists – composed of senior clinicians and forensic psychiatrists – demanded after furious internal debate, that it be withdrawn. A dissenting minority report was written by the most experienced clinician on the working party.

Professor John Morton wrote in the aftermath:

> Note that the [British Psychological] Society's working party was largely made up of people who actually worked on the topic of memory. The Royal College, however, didn't seem to find it necessary to have any experts in the subject – and it showed.

> (Morton, 1998)

Dr Richard Green is an American sexologist, lawyer and psychiatrist, specialising in homosexuality and transsexualism, author of *The Sissy Boy Syndrome* (Green, 1987). In 2002 he argued that paedophilia should not be classified by the American Psychiatric Association as a mental disorder, without impinging on the legal and law enforcement aspects.

In 2010 he wrote a frontispiece and back-cover puff for Carl Toms' book *Dangerous Liaisons* about Michael Jackson. Toms is a pseudonym for Tom O'Carroll, the convicted former leader of the Paedophile Information Exchange (PIE), who has more recently, in 2015, been given a further suspended sentence for indecent assault and gross indecency against two brothers aged 9 and 10 to which he pled guilty.

Green writes of the book:

> the writer promotes an alternative view of boy-man sexuality. It can be, he contends, mutually positive. It can be more than sexual – caring, bonding, loving ... whether or not one is convinced, shaken or even stirred by the author, this is a recommended read.

> (Toms, 2010)

Two other prominent False Memory Syndrome Foundation Advisory Board members are Professors Elizabeth Loftus and Richard Ofshe. Loftus is a respected academic psychologist whose much-quoted laboratory experiment of successfully implanting a fictitious childhood memory of being lost in a shopping mall is much used to defend the FMS argument. In the experiment, older family members persuaded younger ones of the (supposedly) never real event. However, Loftus herself says being lost, which almost everyone has experienced, is in no way similar to being abused. Jennifer Freyd comments on the shopping mall experiment in *Betrayal Trauma*: "If this demonstration proves to hold up under replication it suggests both that therapists can induce false memories and, even more directly, that older family members play a powerful role in defining reality for dependent younger family members" (Freyd, 1996).

Elizabeth Loftus herself was sexually abused as a child by a male babysitter and admits to blacking the perpetrator out of her memory, although she never forgot the incident. In her autobiography *Witness for the Defense* she talks of experiencing flashbacks of this abusive incident on occasion in court (Loftus, 1992). In her teens, having been told by an uncle that she had found her mother's drowned body, she then started to visualise the scene. Her brother later told her that she had not.

Professor Loftus's successful academic career has run parallel to her even more high-profile career as an expert witness in court, for the defence of those accused of rape, murder and child abuse. She is described in her own book as the expert who puts memory on trial. She used her theories on the unreliability of memory to cast doubt on the testimony of the only eye witness left alive who could identify Ted Bundy, the all-American boy, who was one of America's worst serial rapists and killers (Loftus, 1992). Notwithstanding Loftus's arguments the judge kept Bundy in prison. He was eventually tried, convicted and executed.

Loftus resigned from the American Psychological Association in 1996, claiming it had become unscientific. She says she had no knowledge of two ethics complaints that had been filed a month prior with the APA by Lynn Crook and Jennifer Hoult, two abuse survivors who had separately won court cases against their fathers. In both instances there was corroborating evidence additional to their recovered memories. They claim that Loftus had misrepresented their cases in print and in quotes (Treating Abuse Today, 1992).

Professor Richard Ofshe, Professor of Sociology at Berkeley University, California, was also a high-profile spokesman for the concept of "false memory". Like Elizabeth Loftus, he has been an expert witness in court, renowned for having experimentally "implanted" a false memory in the Paul Ingrams case to prove that such a thing was possible. In 1990, Appellate Judge Robert H. Peterson reviewed the testimony and evidence of the case. In his summation, he remarked that Ofshe was neither a clinical psychologist, nor an expert in sex abuse. He described Ofshe's implanting experiment as "odd in my judgement" given that Ofshe gave Ingrams "a false set of facts, but a set of facts that came pretty close to what one of the victims had accused the defendant of". The judge refused to set aside Ingrams' guilty pleas, subsequent appeals have been turned down, and he remained in jail (Peterson, 1990).

Richard Ofshe was ruled inadmissible as an expert witness in a previous case where he had appeared for the defendant who claimed he committed mail frauds as a result of being "brainwashed" by the Church of Scientology. The court ruling states that Dr Ofshe was not "a mental health professional, his testimony was not relevant to the issues, his theories regarding thought reform are not generally accepted within the scientific community ..." (Burgess, 1994; Olio & Cornell, 1994; USA vs. Fishman, 1990).

Richard Ofshe is described in his book as a "joint Pulitzer Prize winner" but the Pulitzer Prize Office at Columbia University has been obliged to issue a statement that he does not appear on any Pulitzer citation (Letter, 1996).

Another key figure in the FMS movement is New Zealand doctor, Felicity Goodyear-Smith. Her book *First Do No Harm* is subtitled "The Sexual Abuse Industry" (Goodyear-Smith, 1993). It is recommended as "excellent" in the British FMS review which applauds the author's attempts to downplay what it describes as misplaced professional over-concern about sexual abuse. The reviewer in the BFMS Newsletter, Ivan Tyrrell, says "her arguments offer a scientific and rational perspective backed by substantial studies and research" in contrast to the hysteria, outrage and ideological beliefs of the "sexual abuse industry" (Tyrrell, 1994).

The major theme in *First Do No Harm* is that sexual abuse is a cultural taboo. There is no intrinsic moral objection to adult–child sexual contact and no automatic damage caused by it. Underwager and Wakefield are quoted as the principal references.

Felicity Goodyear-Smith admits to a personal as well as professional involvement in the abuse field. Her husband and parents-in-law were imprisoned for sexual abuse offences, having been members of a New Zealand community, CentrePoint, which encouraged sexual intimacy amongst its members, including the children.

The author quotes studies that purport to show that adult–child sex can be harmless. Under a section on "Children's Sexual Rights" she describes groups, such as the Paedophile Information Exchange, the Rene Guyon Society ("sex by eight, or it's too late"), and the North American Man/Boy Love Association, as "holding radical beliefs regarding children's sexual rights". She further says, "As would be expected, these societies have mostly been disbanded or outlawed in the sexually repressive 1980s and 1990s".

The studies quoted are by Theo Sandfort and Baurmann. Sandfort was a board member of *Paedika* – the Dutch paedophile magazine and his study consisted of interviewing 25 boys who were recruited by their current adult lovers through a Netherlands paedophile network (Sandfort, 1983). They "demonstrated" to his satisfaction that sexual friendships between men and boys produced no evidence of harm. The Baurmann study is presented as assessing 8058 young people and finding that not one of the 1000 boys under 14 was found to be harmed. In fact, only 112 were sampled for symptoms and of those only 13 were boys, and they tended to be victims of less serious and extra-familial abuse (Baurmann, 1983).

Goodyear-Smith emphasises that the allegations of child abuse in the Australian Children of God sect were unfounded. The age of sexual consent, she thinks is unenforceable and should be removed from the statute books. On her website she argues against mandatory reporting of child abuse (www.goodyearsmith.com).

Conclusion: No one doubts that memory is fallible, subject to distortion, but a considerable number of studies indicate dissociative amnesia occurs and that a majority of recovered memories can be corroborated from outside sources. There were several reasons why the "false memory" media campaign gained traction. One was the libel risk, which prevented journalists from covering both sides of the story. Accused parents could and did speak publicly with little fear of repercussion from their adult children; the reverse was not the case. Where professionals were involved, doctors or psychotherapists, they were ethically bound to confidentiality so could not correct errors of fact. The public had also become satiated by the flood of sexual abuse stories emerging in the late 1980s and found the denial story more palatable.

A sociology study by Katherine Beckett of the University of Michigan looking at USA media coverage of sexual abuse found that in 1991, more than 80% of the coverage was weighted towards stories of survivors, with recovered memory taken for granted and questionable therapy virtually ignored. By 1994 more than 80% of the coverage focussed on false accusation, often involving supposedly false memory. Beckett credited the False Memory Syndrome Foundation with a major role in the change (Beckett, 1996).

What was not generally understood was that the "Memory Wars" were fuelled in part by a science argument, with eminent professionals on the advisory boards defending theories which did not account for the burgeoning evidence of dissociative amnesia. The major psychiatric, psychological and psychotherapy organisations were also slow to find a voice and allowed themselves to be damaged by their late response to the "false memory" argument, by which time it had become common currency.

References

Accuracy About Abuse Newsletter (2 June 1994; AAA10 March 1996).

Baurmann, M.C. (1983). Sexualitat, Gewalt und psychische Folgen. *Wisebaden: Bundeskriminalamt, Forschungsreihe (Sexuality, Violence and Psychic Impact)*, 15.

Beckett, K. (1 February 1996). Culture and the Politics of Signification: The Case of Child Sexual Abuse. *Social Problems*, 43 (1), 57–76.

Bickerton, D. (26 January 1997). Book Review. *New York Times*.

Freyd, W. (17 April1995). Letter to WGBH-Boston.

Freyd, J. (August 1993). *Theoretical and personal perspectives on the delayed memory debate*. Public Lecture, Ann Arbor, reprinted in *Treating Abuse Today*, 3 (5).

Freyd, J. (1996). *Betrayal Trauma: The Logic of Forgetting Childhood Abuse*. Cambridge, MA: Harvard University Press, p. 104.

Freyd, J. & Birrell, P. (2013). *Blind to Betrayal*. London: John Wiley & Sons.

Goodyear-Smith, F. (1993). *First Do No Harm*. New Zealand: Benton-Guy Publishing.

Goodyear-Smith, F. (n.d.). www.goodyearsmith.com.

Geraci, J. (1993). Interview: Hollida Wakefield and Ralph Underwager. *Paidika*, 3 (2), 2–12.

Geraci, J. (May 1997). *Dares to Speak*. London: Gay Men's Press.

Green, R. (1987). *The Sissy Boy Syndrome*. London: Yale University Press.

Kitzinger, J. (1998). The Gender Politics of News Production: Silenced Voices and False Memories. In C. Carter *et al.* (Eds.), *News Gender and Power*. London: Routledge

Letter: The Pulitzer Prizes. (1 May 1996). Office of the Administrator.

Loftus, E. (1992). *Witness for the Defense*. New York: St. Martin's Press, pp. 149, 61–91.

Morton, J., Andrews, B., Bekerian, D., Brewin, C., Davies, G. & Mollon, P. (1995). Recovered Memories: The Report of the Working Party of the British Psychological Society. Leicester: British Psychological Society.

Morton, John. (August 1998). *The Psychologist*, 408.

Observer. (14 May 1995). Life, 6.

Olio, K. & Cornell, W. (1994) The Facade of Scientific Documentation: A Case Study of Richard Ofshe's Analysis of the Paul Ingram Case. (In press: *J. of Interpersonal Violence*).

Salter, A. (1991). Accuracy of Expert testimony in Child Sexual Abuse Cases. A Case study of Ralph Underwager and Hollida Wakefield. Unpublished manuscript on file with the American Prosecutors Research Institute, National Center for Prosecution of Child Abuse (Alexandria, VA).

Stanton, M. (July/August 1997). U Turn on Memory Lane. *Columbia Journalism Review*, 44–49.

Toms, C. (May 2010) *Michael Jackson Dangerous Liaisons*. Leicester: Troubadour Publishing.

Treating Abuse Today. (1996). Vol 5, No. 6/Vol 6, No. 1, 71–73. Ethics Complaints Filed against Prominent FMSF Board Member.

Paul Ross Ingram v Chase Riverland. (1994). No C93–5399FDB Burgess, F. Motion for summary judgement.

Peterson, T. (1990). State of Washington vs Paul Ross Ingram. Superior Court of the state of Washington in and for the county of Thurston, Proceedings, Vol. V11, No. 88-1-752-1.

Sandfort. T. (1983). Pedophile relationships in Netherlands: alternative lifestyle for children? *Alternative Lifestyles*, 5 (3), 164–183.

Tyrrell, I. (10 December 1994). Untitled (Review of *First Do No Harm*). *BFMS Newsletter*, 2 (3).

Underwager and Wakefield v. Salter et al. (1994). No. 93–2422 (W.D. Wisconsin).

USA v Fishman. (13 April 1990). No CR-88–0616-DL (US District Court for Northern District of California).

Chapter 3

The rocky road to false memories

Stories the media missed

Lynn Crook

Adults molested as children spoke out publicly in the mid-1980s and soon gained the right to sue for damages. Accused parents responded by reframing incest allegations as false memories. The parents spent $7M on a campaign in the 1990s directed to the popular press and textbook editors where their claims remain unchallenged.

The *Boston Globe*'s investigative approach to the story of the Catholic Church transferring priests who were accused of molesting children resulted in a Pulitzer. These multi-victim accusations against priests were considered corroborated cases. Rather than relying on the accused priests and their experts for their story as the media had done in the 1990s for single-victim cases, reporters did their homework. The investigative approach continued as reporters uncovered long-standing institutional tolerance of multi-victim child molesters in churches, private schools, universities, gymnastic and scouting organisations.

As shown in the 2018 media coverage of Christine Blasey Ford's accusation of teenage sexual assault, many in the media default to false memories in covering single-victim accusations. Therefore, it is important that we understand why and how the false memory scenario was adopted by the media.

When a jury found George Franklin guilty in 1990 of the murder of 8-year-old Susan Nason based upon the recovered memories of his daughter, Eileen Franklin, the media covered the story (People v. Franklin, 1990). In 1991, *People Magazine* featured cover stories of three celebrities who recovered memories of childhood incest. Actress Sandra Dee (Dee, 1991) was on a March cover, former Miss America Marilyn van Derbur Atler (Atler, 1991) appeared in June and television star Roseanne Barr (Arnold, 1991) was on the October cover. The three women, role models for their many fans, described how they recalled molestation by their fathers. Dee recalled on her wedding night, Atler in a conversation with a long-time friend, and Barr during a phone call. The women discussed the consequences of the abuse. They told their own stories. Experts were not called upon to interpret their stories.

By 1991 nearly two dozen US state legislatures had passed laws allowing adults who were molested as children to sue for damages based on recovered memories, or on a recent realisation of the damage caused by the abuse. The

DOI: 10.4324/9781003193159-4

old defences, "My hand slipped", "She seduced me", "I was drunk" or "Some other dude did it (SODDI)", would not stand up under cross-examination in these lawsuits. A new defence was needed.

Elizabeth Loftus was a psychology professor at the University of Washington with a second profession. She provided research and expert testimony for the defence to counter eyewitness testimony in criminal cases. She was called upon to testify for the defence in the Franklin murder trial. She also testified for the defence in Patti Barton's lawsuit (Barton v. Peters, 1990) against her father after Barton had lobbied for a law extending the statute of limitations for such claims. Loftus's testimony failed to prevail in both cases.

Loftus tossed out ideas for a new defence in 1991 for those facing long-ago molestation charges. Repressed memories are "suspicious", she told *Toronto Star* reporter Marilyn Dunlop in February (Dunlop, 1991). "Are the accusations driven by hatred and revenge?" Loftus asked *Seattle Post–Intelligencer* reporter Judi Hunt in May (Hunt, 1991).

In August, Loftus suggested to Tracy Thompson at the *Washington Post*, "An overly zealous psychologist could unwittingly use his or her influence over a vulnerable patient to plant the seeds of a 'memory' that is actually a fantasy". The *Post* dropped "fantasy" from the scenario, then elevated the theory to headline status as "Delayed Lawsuits of Sexual Abuse on the Rise; Alleged Victims Base Legal Actions on Memories Critics Say May Be Implanted in Therapy" (Thompson, 1991).

Parents accused of long-ago sexual abuse now had their defence – the accusations were implanted by therapists. In Elizabeth Loftus, the parents had a world-renowned researcher who would point out to reporters as well as to judges and juries the suggestive influences in each case that might have resulted in false memories.

The False Memory Syndrome Foundation opened for business in March 1992. The group presented a new approach on child sexual abuse to the media. The adults who claimed to be molested as children were, in fact, the victims of manipulative therapists who implanted these memories.

Could therapists, in fact, implant entire memories of childhood molestation in their clients? To determine whether this was possible, Loftus offered her fall quarter 1991 cognitive psychology students an extra credit assignment: Design a method to make someone believe they were lost in a shopping mall as a child. The implication in this assignment was that the trauma of getting lost in a shopping mall was similar to that of being sexually abused by one's parent. The assumption was also made that if an older relative who had supposedly witnessed the getting lost incident could convince a younger relative they were lost, then a therapist who did not witness the molestation of a client could convince a client they were molested as a child. Loftus's student, undergrad James Coan, came up with four stories about his younger brother. Three were true. The fourth story implied Coan was present when his younger brother at age 5 allegedly got lost at the University City Mall in Spokane. Coan's mother and his brother repeated the stories for five days. Coan's mother said she didn't recall her younger son getting lost; Coan's brother reported a specific, elaborated memory of getting lost at the mall. Coan had his five extra credit points. Loftus had a story for the media. Coan's story was received by the media as a valid scientific experiment, even though it was a class exercise and not sanctioned by the university's Human Subjects Committee.

Reporters appeared impressed with Coan's false memory "experiment". Psychologist Dan Goleman, PhD, a reporter at the *New York Times* called Coan's success, "A pertinent experiment on the malleability of human memory". Goleman informed readers about the False Memory Syndrome Foundation in Philadelphia (Goleman, 1992).

Seattle Times reporter Bill Dietrich's story went out on the Associated Press newswire establishing a copy-editing standard – sneer quotes around "repressed": "UW Expert Challenges 'Repressed' Memories – Says Some Sexual Abuse May Not Be Real" (Dietrich, 1992).

Goleman and Dietrich as well as the dozens of reporters who followed failed to note that Coan's methodology as well as in the methodology of the formal mall study that followed did not parallel what a therapist might say to a client.

Some have suggested the media's failure to challenge the false memory scenario reflected a need to deny the scale of the sexual abuse of children. Perhaps their editors failed to encourage a critical analysis of the story because everyone else was covering it – so it must be true. Some reporters may have failed to question the story because they had been accused of molesting a child. Others may have been protecting someone. Some may have been hoping for a Pulitzer. And some reporters may have been influenced by psychology textbooks that gave extensive coverage to the deficits of memory and the false memory debate, another successful objective accomplished by the False Memory Syndrome Foundation (Brand & McEwen, 2014).

Whatever the reason, reporters listened, they took notes and they headed off to write their stories. By 1994 85% of the media coverage of adults' accusations of childhood sex abuse focused on false memories (Beckett, 1996). Meanwhile, the archive of corroborated recovered memory cases at http://blogs.brown.edu/recoveredmemory/case-archive/, and the annotated bibliography of research corroborating recovered memories at http://www.leadershipcouncil.org/1/tm/amnesia.html received no press coverage. Thirty-four media representatives attended the Foundation's first conference in Valley Forge in April 1993: ABC, CBS, Fox, NBC News, CBC TV, Blue Sky Productions, *Answers in Action Journal, Changes Magazine, Family Therapy Networker, Insight Magazine, Moving Forward,* Mother Jones, *The New Yorker, The Philadelphia Inquirer, Psychology Today* and the *San Diego Union-Tribune* (FMSF, May 1993). Reporters sat and listened as future American Psychological Association president Martin Seligman introduced a panel of Foundation board members. Judge Lisa Richette from Philadelphia chaired the "What Do Lawyers Need?" panel, and Judge Phyllis W. Beck from the Superior Court of Pennsylvania chaired "Did the Crime Occur?" (FMSF, March 1993).

The story presented at the Foundation's conference was not about middle-class accused parents selling their new defence to the media. Instead, the media reported stories of families torn apart by memories implanted by inept therapists. As the media focused on false accusations in 1994, Loftus's lost in the mall study, intended to show that false memories can be implanted, appeared to be in trouble.

Dan Goleman at the *New York Times* quoted the final mall study result which Loftus announced at a conference:

> About 10 percent (2 subjects) of adults will come up with a specific elaborated memory from childhood, and another 15 percent (3 subjects) or so will say they feel a vague sense of certainty that it occurred if you keep asking them about it.
>
> (Goleman, 1994)

Loftus's final report to the Human Subjects Committee states, "8–9% have formed false positive memories. Another 10–15% formed partial false memories" (Human Subjects Review Committee, 1994). "Partial" memories meant the subjects had remembered something about the incident (the subjects had, in fact, visited that mall with family members) or they had speculated about how and when it may have happened (p. 722). With 2 of the 24 subjects reporting "a specific elaborated memory", opposing attorneys would easily dismiss the result as "just lucky guesses". Recent reviews of the mall study found that not only did the mall study not relate to what a therapist might say, but all of the 24 subjects apparently correctly identified the lost in a mall story as false (Crook & McEwen, 2019; Blizzard & Shaw, 2019).

The road to false memories for abuse allegations appeared to be getting rocky in 1995. When the mall study was published in Psychiatric Annals in December 1995, the result (p. 723) had been increased from two subjects to five subjects (Loftus & Pickrell, 1995). Loftus faced additional "misrepresentation" problems in 1995 beyond the failed mall study. The APA journal, *Clinical Psychology*, released Koss, Tromp & Tharan (1995) reporting that the data in "Mental Shock Can Produce Retrograde Amnesia" (Loftus & Burns, 1982) failed to support the authors' conclusion.

Two ethics complaints were filed against Loftus in December 1995. Both complainants had successfully sued for damages based on recovered memories. Both complainants (this author and Jennifer Hoult) claimed Loftus had misrepresented their cases to the media. The complaints were not investigated after Loftus faxed her resignation to the APA a few weeks later, on 16 January 1996, claiming APA activities "have moved in directions that are disturbingly far from scientific thinking". Neither the Koss et al. (1995) article nor the ethics complaints stories were covered by the popular press.

With its membership beginning to slow after reaching just over 2000 members in 1994, the Foundation turned its attention to another issue – filing ethics complaints and lawsuits against therapists. PBS Frontline producer Ofra Bikel's "The Search for Satan" in 1995 (https://www.pbs.org/wgbh/frontline/film/the-search-for-satan/) featured Pat Burgus and Mary Shanley. Both women had sued their therapists for malpractice (Burgus v. Braun, 1997; Shanley v. Braun, 1997), claiming their memories of childhood abuse were implanted. Reviewers praised the programme. On 17 January 1997 Burgus conceded in her deposition that, other than what she had recalled herself, her psychiatrist, Braun, MD, had told her only what other patients were saying about her (pp. 912–13). No memories were implanted. The memory implanting issue was not made public since the lawsuit was settled, despite Braun's contractual right to go to trial. Burgus and her sons settled for a record-breaking $10.6 million in late October 1997. The media covered the story of the settlement.

Mary Shanley became the government's star witness in a federal case in Houston after a grand jury in 1997 indicted Judith A. Peterson, PhD, Richard E. Seward, MD, George Jerry Mueck, Gloria Keraga, MD, and Sylvia Davis, MSW, on conspiracy and fraud charges (United States v. Peterson et al., 1999). If found guilty, the defendants would spend the rest of their lives in prison for diagnosing a dissociative disorder and billing through the mail for treatment.

The government's witnesses included many of the individuals who had appeared in Frontline producer Ofra Bikel's "The Search for Satan". In court, their stories did not hold up as well as they had in Bikel's interviews. Under cross-examination by Peterson's attorney, Rusty Hardin, Shanley conceded on 8 October 1997 that she could not name any memories that were implanted. The *Houston Chronicle* headline on 8 October 1998 announced, "Former patient can't attribute false memories to therapy" (Smith, 1999). On 1 March 1999 the government moved to dismiss the indictment. The national media did not cover the story.

Reporters faithfully attended FMS Foundation conferences until 2002 when a new story made headlines. The false memory approach to sex abuse allegations faded as the *Boston Globe*'s Spotlight investigative team uncovered widespread multi-victim priest abuse cases in the Boston area. The priests had been transferred following the accusations. The *Globe* received a Pulitzer in 2003. Another Pulitzer was awarded to Sara Ganim at the *Patriot News* in 2012 for her story on the Penn State multi-victim abuse scandal involving former football coach Jerry Sandusky.

Reporters did not contact false memory experts for their "take" on these multi-victim accusations. False memories also did not play a role in #MeToo coverage of multi-victim sexual harassment by men in positions of power. Instead, we heard from the women who were assaulted. So too with the media coverage of Dr Larry Nassar, the former team USA Gymnastics doctor who molested more than 200 gymnasts. False memory experts did not interpret these stories for us. We listened in 2018 as the young women he assaulted told their own stories.

Reporters returned to false memory speculation once again in their coverage of a single-victim disclosure in September 2018. As Christine Blasey Ford prepared to testify before the Senate in September 2018 regarding her accusation of sexual assault against Supreme Court nominee Brett Kavanaugh, reporters either interviewed Elizabeth Loftus, or they quoted an earlier online statement.

Following the decade-long false memory campaign initiated by middle-class parents accused of incest, the media has remained sceptical of individual adults' allegations of childhood sexual abuse. The media have failed to note that the research supporting false memory claims does not apply to what a therapist might conceivably say to a client. The public's largely sceptical response to disclosures of childhood sexual abuse by family members and friends reflects the media's scepticism. After nearly 30 years perhaps the time has come for us to take a critical look at the impact of the false memory campaign on the media and on our culture.

References

Arnold, R. (7 October1991). A Star Cries Incest. *People.* https://people.com/archive/cover-story-a-star-cries-incest-vol-36-no-13/

Atler, M. V. (10 June1991). The Darkest Secret. *People.* https://people.com/archive/cover-story-the-darkest-secret-vol-35-no-22/

Barton v. Peters. (1990). 4FA-90–0157 (Superior Court for the State of Alaska, 4th Judicial District).

Beckett, K. (1996). Culture and the Politics of Signification: The Case of Child Sexual Abuse. *Social Problems,* 43 (1), 57–76.

Blizzard, R. A. & Shaw, M. (2019). Lost-in-the-Mall: False Memory or False Defense? *Journal of Child Custody.* doi:10.1080/15379418.2019.1590285

Brand, B. L. & McEwen, L. E. (Fall, 2014). Coverage of Child Maltreatment and its Effects in Three Introductory Psychology Textbooks. *Trauma Psychology News,* Division 56 of the American Psychology Association, pp. 8–11. http://traumapsychnews.com/archived-issues/#2014

Burgus v. Braun. (1997). 91L8493/91L8493 (Circuit Court, Cook County, Illinois).

Crook, L. & McEwen, L. (2019). Deconstructing the Lost in the Mall Study. *Journal of Child Custody,* 16 (1), 7–19.

Dee, S. (18 March1991). Learning to Live Again. *People.* https://people.com/archive/cover-story-learning-to-live-again-vol-35-no-10/

Dietrich, B. (13 August1992). UW Expert Challenges "Repressed" Memories – Says Some Sexual Abuse May Not Be Real. *Seattle Times.* http://tinyurl.com/ha949lv

Dunlop, M. (25 February1991). Playing Tricks With Your Memory. *Toronto Star,* 2C. http://pqasb.pqarchiver.com/thestar/access/461648651.html?dids=461648651:4616486 51&FMT=ABS&FMTS=ABS:FT&type=current&date=Feb+25%2C+1991&author=Marilyn+Dunlop+TORONTO+STAR&pub=Toronto+Star&desc=Playing+tricks+with+your+memory+Mind+can+be+manipulated%2C+pro

FMS Foundation Newsletter (FMSF) (1993), *FMSF Newsletter Archive.* http://www.fmsfonline.org

Goleman, D. (21 July1992). Childhood Trauma: Memory or Invention? *New York Times.* https://www.nytimes.com/1992/07/21/science/childhood-trauma-memory-or-invention.html

Goleman, D. (31 May1994). Miscoding is Seen as the Root of False Memories. *New York Times*. https://www.nytimes.com/1994/05/31/science/miscoding-is-seen-as-the-root-of-false-memories.html?pagewanted=all

Human Subjects Review Committee. (1994). Status Report Application #23–332-C (1 June 1994). *Review of Experiment involving Human Subjects*. University of Washington.

Hunt, J. (2 May1991). Just Memories: Psychologist States the Case Against "Infallible" Witnesses. *Seattle Post–Intelligencer*, D1.

Koss, M., Tromp, S. & Tharan, M. (Summer, 1995). Traumatic Memories: Empirical Foundations, Forensic and Clinical Implications. *Clinical Psychology: Science and Practice*, 2 (2), 111–131.

Loftus, E. & Burns, T. (1982). Mental Shock Can Produce Retrograde Amnesia. *Memory & Cognition*, 10, 318–323.

Loftus, E. & Pickrell, J. (1995). The Formation of False Memories. *Psychiatric Annals*, 25, 720–725. http://users.ecs.soton.ac.uk/harnad/Papers/Py104/loftus.mem.html

People v. Franklin. (30 November1990). C-24395 (San Mateo County Superior Court).

Smith, M. (October 9 1998). Former Patient Can't Attribute False Memories to Therapy. *Houston Chronicle*.

Shanley v. Braun. (1997). WL 779112 (N.D. Ill.).

Thompson, T. (14 August1991). Delayed Lawsuits of Sexual Abuse on the Rise; Alleged Victims Base Legal Actions On Memories Critics Say May Be Implanted in Therapy. *The Washington Post*. https://www.highbeam.com/doc/1P2-1079806.html

United States v. Peterson. (6 October1999). 71 F. Supp. 2d 695 (US District Court for the Southern District of Texas).

Chapter 4

Re-examining the "Lost in the Mall" study

Were "false memories" created to promote a false defence? In conversation with Ruth Blizard

Valerie Sinason

In this interview, Ruth Blizard lays bare in stark detail the false premises of the "Lost in the Mall" study by Elizabeth Loftus. This study has been one of the major pillars on which false memory societies all over the world have erected their false defences against adults' memories. In examining the ethics, the non-science and the use made of this faulty paper, Blizard dismantles the false defence made from it.

VALERIE: You have spoken powerfully of the concept of false memory as a "false defence". Can you explain the original legal context of your phrase?

RUTH: The notion that false memories could be readily induced by suggestion was promoted by the False Memory Syndrome Foundation (FMSF) as a defence against adult survivors' testimony that they had been abused by their parents. In cases where survivors had forgotten experiences of abuse, and then remembered again in adulthood, Loftus, and many other "expert witnesses", used the "Lost in the Mall" research (Loftus & Pickrell, 1995) to allege that these memories were implanted by psychotherapists. This became the false memory defence.

I refer to this as a false defence for several reasons:

1   No evidence was presented to demonstrate that full false memories were induced in the "Lost in the Mall" study (Blizard & Shaw, 2019).
2   Believing that one had been lost while shopping in childhood is not analogous to remembering sexual abuse. In fact, a large proportion of subjects can be convinced that they were lost in a mall as children, but none could be led to falsely believe they had been administered enemas (Pezdek, Finger & Hodge, 1997).
3   To date, there are no studies showing that memories can be implanted for repeated events, as is often the case with childhood sexual abuse, nor for intimate relations with family in general. "Nor is there yet evidence to

DOI: 10.4324/9781003193159-5

show that false memories can be created with the degree of conviction necessary to sustain protracted legal proceedings involving the police and cross-examination in the courts" (Brewin & Andrews, 2017, p. 20).

4   The "Lost in the Mall" experimental paradigm depends on an older relative stating that they were present when the subject was lost. Even if a therapist suggests that a patient may have been traumatised, they do not invite trusted family members to convince them that childhood abuse occurred (Andrews & Brewin, 2017).

VALERIE: What are the key scientific flaws in the mall study?

RUTH: The first six subjects in the formal mall study failed to develop false memories (Coan, 1993), but those results were never published. In the second iteration of the formal mall study (Loftus & Pickrell, 1995), there is little explicit description of the methods of recruitment of subjects, experimental controls or training of investigators. The description of methods of rating full and partial false memories is vague, and there is no definition of what constitutes a full memory. Most importantly, no evidence is presented that any subjects formed full false memories. Nevertheless, the authors imply that, based on study results, they "are providing an 'existence proof' for the phenomenon of false memory formation" (pp. 723–4). To the contrary, Loftus had confirmed earlier that the existence proof is based solely on informal observations and anecdotes (Crook v. Murphy, 1994; Loftus & Ketcham, 1994). These were unsupervised trials conducted by Loftus's undergraduate students with their own family members.

VALERIE: What are your main ethical and scientific concerns about the concept of "false memory syndrome"?

RUTH: No experimental studies have demonstrated that full autobiographical memories can be implanted by suggestion. False memory experiments based on the "Lost in the Mall" paradigm deceive subjects by providing evidence from trusted family members. They may come to believe the false story happened, but they are not likely to have a full autobiographical memory of actually experiencing that event (Brewin & Andrews, 2017).

Pezdek and Hinz (2002) re-interpreted the results of the "Lost in the Mall" study (Loftus & Pickrell, 1995). They pointed out that subjects who were considered to have remembered the false event, "simply recalled some of the true information in the description of the false event: that is, the suggested false event was not really planted in memory" (p. 101). Hyman and Pentland (1996) commented, "Suggestions regarding an event do not appear to be adopted wholesale. Rather ... the individual considers the suggestions in light of other ... personal memories ... and constructs a memory that is a combination of the suggestion plus related self-knowledge" (p. 112).

Memory implantation studies use two tactics to persuade subjects to believe that suggested false events are true. First, they use a trusted authority such as a parent or older sibling to provide information about the event to convince subjects it actually occurred. As a result, the subjects may believe it happened to them, even though they do not actually recall being there. Second, subjects often feel social demand to agree with their relative. This may motivate them to retrieve information of similar events from long-term memory. They may then attribute those details to the specific story presented in the study. Loftus and Pickrell (1995) agree that false recall in their study "can be viewed as a form of source confusion", continuing, "Some elements of the false memories created by us … are represented in long-term memory prior to the experiment" (p. 725). Thus, what appear to be full false memories may, in fact, be partially constructed from true elements of similar experiences in autobiographical memory.

VALERIE: How did the False Memory Syndrome Foundation spread bias against abuse survivors in the courts and the media?

RUTH: The FMSF was established in 1991 in response to the increasing recognition and prosecution of child sexual abuse in the 1980s and 1990s. Because new laws allowed adults abused as children to sue for damages, accused parents searched for new means of legal defence that would stand up in court. The FMSF was established to advocate for parents who believed they had been falsely accused by their adult children who had recovered memories of childhood abuse. They denounced these accusations as false memory syndrome (FMS). The mall study was developed in this context (Loftus & Ketcham, 1994), and subsequently the principal investigator, Elizabeth Loftus, used it to provide expert testimony in defence of people accused of child abuse. She soon joined the FMSF Scientific and Professional Advisory Board (Crook & McEwen, 2019).

The FMSF initiated a campaign to convince the public and the legal community that false memories of childhood abuse can be implanted by therapists, because this could be used as a defence by accused parents (Crook & McEwen, 2019). As a result, the conclusion of the mall study, that false memories can be easily implanted by suggestion, has been pervasively cited in legal testimony, psychology textbooks (Wilgus et al., 2016), false memory research (Brewin & Andrews, 2017) and the popular media (Crook & McEwen, 2019).

VALERIE: What do you see as the most dangerous aspect of the early FMSF position?

RUTH: FMS and parental alienation syndrome (PAS) were developed as defences for parents accused of child abuse as part of a larger movement to undermine the prosecution of child abuse. The formation of the FMSF in 1991 was preceded by the founding of Victims of Child Abuse Laws (VOCAL), an advocacy organisation that sought to weaken child protective laws (Cheit, 2014). These societies buttressed the backlash against the recognition and prosecution of child sexual abuse cases in the 1980s and 1990s (Salter, 1998).

VOCAL was founded by expert witness, Ralph Underwager, and some of the 24 defendants he helped to acquit in the Jordan, Minnesota, cases of organised child molestation (Cheit, 2014). In the late 1980s, VOCAL helped defendants accused of child abuse find sympathetic expert witnesses to defend them in court. It may also have served to develop a network of defendants who believed they were falsely accused of child abuse, and, conceivably, many of them may later have joined the FMSF.

VALERIE: How is Parental Alienation Syndrome related to false memory?

RUTH: Before the FMS defence was used to discredit the testimony of adult survivors, parental alienation syndrome (Gardner, 1985, 1998) was used to defend parents accused of abuse in child custody cases. PAS implies that children are highly suggestible and can be coached or "brainwashed" into falsely believing they have been abused. This is purported to cause the children to alienate their affections from the accused parent. Just as the false memory defence calls into question the testimony of adult survivors, the PAS defence undermines the credibility of children's testimony, discredits the protective parents, and persuades judges to dismiss abuse allegations. In fact, children are much more likely to minimise and deny abuse, rather than exaggerate or over-report it (Lawson & Chaffin, 1992; Sjoberg & Lindblad, 2002).

While PAS discredits the testimony of children and protective parents, it all too often allows manipulative abusers to claim they were falsely accused. Research shows that it is most often noncustodial parents (usually fathers) who make intentionally false reports, while custodial parents (usually mothers) and children were least likely to fabricate reports of abuse or neglect (Trocme & Bala, 2005). Nevertheless, PAS has been very successfully used in the family law courts to strip parental rights from the parent alleging child abuse or domestic violence, and reassign custody to the parent being accused. The FMSF went one step further to discredit the testimony of child abuse survivors, by using a research study (Loftus & Pickrell, 1995) to suggest that therapists or forensic interviewers could implant false memories of abuse. A claim of FMS implies there is no basis for an abuse allegation in court. This strategy takes all blame off the child victim and makes it easier for victims under pressure from family members to retract their accusations.

VALERIE: Are the "false memories" generated in research settings true autobiographical memories?

RUTH: The FMSF made it appear as though there was a recognised "syndrome" or mental disorder that causes individuals to believe they experienced childhood events that did not happen. However, there is no evidence that persons can be led to believe falsely that they were abused with sufficient conviction to carry out a protracted court case (Brewin & Andrews, 2017).

Loftus did not provide evidence that any full false memories were produced in her study. However, later false memory studies did find evidence that a minority of subjects could be convinced they experienced something in childhood that didn't happen (e.g. Hyman & Pentland, 1996). Those subjects may have come to believe an event happened, but they did not have a true autobiographical memory. Typically, they accepted an older family member's word that the event took place. In more extreme manipulations of subjects' memories, they were presented with a doctored photograph, in which an image of their face was pasted into an event, such as a hot air balloon ride. The subjects may have accepted the suggestion that they experienced this event, but subjectively they doubted the memory's certainty and any thoughts or images about it were vague. If they had images or recollections that seemed related to the false event, they were likely retrieved from memories of a similar event that actually did happen in childhood (Hyman & Pentland, 1996; Pezdek & Hinz, 2002).

VALERIE: What does it mean that the psychology community has not queried the faulty research in the "Lost in the Mall" experiment?

RUTH: It is disconcerting that so much scientific credence has been given to a study whose scientific method has not been directly critiqued. The mall study was heavily promoted to the media by the FMSF (Crook & McEwen, 2019). Pressure not to publish studies criticising the concept of false memory may have influenced the scope of research. Perhaps this is why false memory research has focused narrowly on preventing unsubstantiated allegations of abuse. Regrettably, the research has neglected the possibility that the testimony of genuine abuse survivors may be wrongly dismissed (Becker-Blease & Freyd, 2017; Pope & Brown, 1996).

This bias in the research appears to have had a chilling effect on the publication of studies that question the capacity to generate false memories (Andrews & Brewin, 2017). It may have also deflected inquiry away from studying how perpetrators interfere with survivors' memories for abuse (Becker-Blease & Freyd, 2017). When Brewin and Andrews (2017) wrote the first comprehensive review of the false memory research in over 20 years, they encountered unusually hostile reactions from journal reviewers. The authors speculated as to whether scientific debate was being suppressed (Andrews & Brewin, 2017).

VALERIE: What does it mean that Bernice Andrews and Chris Brewin faced such an unusual non-scientific response to their work?

RUTH: One of the reviewers suggested that Brewin and Andrews (2017) "appear to have some sort of political or social agenda", contributing to their minimising the false memory findings (Andrews & Brewin, 2017). Ironically, a large proportion of the studies demonstrating the generation of false memories make commentaries about the dangers of false accusations of child abuse. Yet, none of these studies examine the memories of childhood abuse. Nor are they attempting to replicate the process of recovering traumatic memories as it might take place in psychotherapy. Rather, most false memory studies attempt to suggest to subjects that they experienced much more commonplace events, such as getting lost, spilling a bowl of punch, going for a balloon ride, or getting sick after eating eggs. It may be profitable to wonder whether many of the false memory researchers have been swept up in the FMSF campaign to exonerate parents who claim they have been falsely accused. Andrews and Brewin (2017) note that "theoretical rigidity and lack of open dialogue are a particular problem for theories that are rooted in public policy or moral advocacy goals" (p. 48).

One contributor to the chilling effect on scientific debate may have been a series of attacks against the author of a critical examination of one of the most widely cited books on children's testimony, Accusations of Child Sexual Abuse (Wakefield & Underwager, 1988). This book claimed that leading and suggestive questioning could influence the testimony of children with regard to sexual abuse. In 1992, Anna Salter wrote an unpublished report, "Accuracy of expert testimony in child sexual abuse cases: A case study of Ralph Underwager and Hollida Wakefield", criticising numerous inaccuracies in the book. In response, Underwager and Wakefield began a campaign of what may be called harassment and intimidation, including the filing of multiple lawsuits and an ethics charge against Salter with the American Psychological Association.

Salter refused the demands to retract her criticism of the book, and the lawsuits and ethics charges were later dismissed (Salter, 1998; Ralph Underwager and Hollida Wakefield v. Anna Salter, 1994). Nevertheless, her ordeal may have intimidated other authors from publishing similar criticisms.

Other researchers and authors attempting to criticise false memory studies may have been intimidated. Between 1992 and 2017, nearly two dozen psychologists, psychiatrists, attorneys, authors, researchers, journalists, and abuse survivors have been subjected to ad hominem attacks by Loftus (Crook, personal communication, 2019). Those defamed include Ellen Bass, E. Sue Blume, Martha Dean, Laura Brown, Mary Harvey, Jim Coan's mother, Judith Herman, David Calof, Kenneth Pope, David Corwin, Diana Russell, Lynn Crook, Lenore Walker, Laura Davis, Charles Whitfield, B. J. Levy, Neil Brick, Karen Olio, Bessel van der Kolk, Holly Ramona, Nicole Taus Kluemper and Gerald Koocher.

VALERIE: How do you feel the professional field should deal with suppression of free speech and scientific inquiry?

RUTH: Sunlight and transparency may be the best antidote to suppression of free inquiry. Bias affecting scientific discourse is nothing new. Forty years ago, empirical evidence showed that reviewers' evaluations are biased according to whether the study's results support their own theoretical position (Mahoney, 1977, cited in Andrews & Brewin, 2017). Failure to publish negative results also distorts what becomes accepted truth.

Recently, there has been renewed interest in re-examining seminal studies. Some, like the Robber's Cave or Stanford prison experiments, have been exposed for suppressing negative results. As a result, long-accepted views on human nature are being called into question. The mall study has shaped the field of false memory research, despite the fact that it presents no evidence of full false memories.

Child abuse is a horrifying phenomenon, and it is natural for people to want to believe that it doesn't exist. Freud apparently succumbed to that form of denial, and, apparently, this was not merely to escape censure by his colleagues (Blizard, 2003). His own diaries suggest he may have been seeking to avoid having to face his own history of abuse (Kupfersmid, 1992). His letters to Fliess indicate that he did not want to believe that his own father could be a perpetrator (Gay, 1989).

Many academics may be equally motivated to deny the existence of child abuse as was Freud. Those who gain considerable income from testifying in defence of accused perpetrators, as have Underwager, Gardner and Loftus, may have additional motivation for claiming that abuse accusations were fabricated.

Changing cultural beliefs and attitudes takes a long time, especially when addressing shocking and painful issues. Academics, clinicians, and advocates for survivors should not be afraid to open up old studies and critique scientific and ethical flaws. It took close to a hundred years to overturn Freud's contention that his patients' memories of abuse were fantasies. It has been nearly a quarter of a century since Loftus claimed false memories of childhood could be readily generated by suggestion, and the FMSF used this finding to profess that therapists could implant false memories of child abuse.

References

Andrews, B. & Brewin, C. R. (2017). False Memories and Free Speech: Is Scientific Debate Being Suppressed? *Applied Cognitive Psychology*, 31, 45–49. doi:10.1002/acp.3285

Becker-Blease, K. & Freyd, J. J. (2017). Additional Questions About the Applicability of "False Memory" Research. *Applied Cognitive Psychology*, 31, 34–36. doi:10.1002/acp.3266

Blizard, R. A. (2003). Why Was Dissociation Dissociated in Psychoanalysis? *Journal of Trauma and Dissociation*, 4 (3), 27–50.

Blizard, R. A. & Shaw, M. (2019). Lost-in-the-Mall: False Memory or False Defense? *Journal of Child Custody*. doi:10.1080/15379418.2019.1590285

Brewin, C. R. & Andrews, B. (2017). Creating Memories for False Autobiographical Events in Childhood: A Systematic Review. *Applied Cognitive Psychology*, 31, 2–23. doi:10.1002/acp.3220

Cheit, R. E. (2014). *The Witch-Hunt Narrative: Politics, Psychology, and the Sexual Abuse of Children*. New York: Oxford University Press.

Coan, J. A. (1993). Creating False Memories. Senior paper, University of Washington, Psychology Honors Program.

Crook, L. S. (2019). Personal communication, references for attacks available from the author.

Crook, L. S. & McEwen, L. E. (2019). Deconstructing the Lost in the Mall Study. *Journal of Child Custody*. doi:10.1080.15379418.2019.1601603

Crook v. Murphy. (1994). Deposition of Elizabeth Loftus in the Matter of Crook v. Murphy, 91-2-01102-5 (Superior Court of the State of Washington, County of Benton24 January1994).

Gardner, R. A. (1985). Recent Trends in Divorce and Custody Litigation. *Academy Forum*, 29 (2), 3–7. http://fact.on.ca/Info/pas/gardnr85.pdf.

Gardner, R. A. (1998). *The Parental Alienation Syndrome* (2nd ed.). Cresskill: Creative Therapeutics.

Gay, P. (1989). *The Freud Reader*. New York: W. W. Norton.

Hyman, I. E., Jr. & Pentland, J. (1996). The Role of Mental Imagery in the Creation Of False Childhood Memories. *Journal of Memory and Language*, 35, 101–117.

Kupfersmid, J. (1992), The "Defence" of Sigmund Freud. *Psychotherapy*, 29 (2), 297–309.

Lawson, L. & Chaffin, M. (1992). False Negatives in Sexual Abuse Disclosure Interviews. *Journal of Interpersonal Violence*, 7 (4), 532–542.

Loftus, E. F. & Ketcham, K. (1994). *The Myth of Repressed Memory: False Memories and Allegations of Sexual Abuse*. New York: St. Martin's Press.

Loftus, E. F. & Pickrell, J. E. (1995). The Formation of False Memories. *Psychiatric Annals*, 25, 720–725.

Pezdek, K., Finger, K. & Hodge, D. (1997). Planting False Childhood Memories: The Role of Event Plausibility. *Psychological Science*, 8 (6), 437–441. https://www.jstor.org/stable/40063230?seq=1#page_scan_tab_contents

Pezdek, K. & Hinz, T. (2002). *The Construction of False Events in Memory*. In H. L. Westcott, G. M. Davies & R. H. C. Bull (Eds.), *Children's Testimony*. New York: John Wiley & Sons.

Pope, Ken S. & Brown, Laura S. (1996). *Recovered Memories of Abuse: Assessment, Therapy, Forensics*. Washington, DC: American Psychological Association.

Ralph Underwager and Hollida Wakefield v. Anna Salter. (1994). 22 F.3d 730 (7th Cir. 1994).

Salter, A. C. (1998). Confessions of a Whistle-Blower: Lessons Learned. *Ethics & Behavior*, 8 (2), 115–124. doi:10.1207/s15327019eb0802_2

Sjoberg, R. L. & Lindblad, F. (2002). Limited Disclosure of Sexual Abuse in Children Whose Experiences Were Documented by Videotape. *American Journal of Psychiatry*, 159 (2), 312–314.

Trocme, N. & Bala, N. (2005). False Allegations of Abuse and Neglect When Parents Separate. *Child Abuse & Neglect*, 29 (12), 1333.

Wakefield, H. & Underwager, R. (1988). *Accusations of Child Sexual Abuse*. Springfield: Charles Thomas.

Wilgus, S. J., Packer, M. M., Lile-King, R., Miller-Perrin, C. L. & Brand, B. L. (2016). Coverage of Child Maltreatment in Abnormal Psychology Textbooks: Reviewing the Adequacy of the Content. *Psychological Trauma: Theory, Research, Practice, & Policy*, 8 (2), 188–197. doi:10.1037/tra0000049

Chapter 5

Evaluating false memory research

Winja Buss

This chapter will introduce three important false memory research paradigms and then go on to outline three important criteria for evaluating false memory research. These criteria help to assess false memory research scientifically. Careful analysis of the research shows it is not easy to implant false memories of childhood abuse. False memories with autobiographical belief, recollective experiences and confidence in memory are rare to non-existent.

Research paradigms

Our memory is undeniably fallible. Memory research is extremely interesting and varied, while only a small branch deals with deliberately implanted false memories. Brewin and Andrews (2016) have conducted a meta-analysis to extract scientific criteria with which we can better understand and evaluate this kind of research. Basically, three experimental paradigms are used to attempt the implantation of false memories in subjects:

Imagination inflation

Subjects are prompted to repeatedly imagine events that never happened, as vividly as possible.

False feedback

Subjects are supplied with false information that suggest the false event has actually happened.

Memory implantation

Subjects are told of corroboration of the false event, i.e. relatives have supposedly confirmed it happened, or subjects are being shown manipulated photographs.

Most studies that combine all three paradigms claim practical relevance with regard to memories of childhood abuse, while omitting critical limitations:

DOI: 10.4324/9781003193159-6

- Definition and operationalisation of "false memories" vary significantly across different studies.
- Differentiating between true and false memories requires a highly complex evaluation process.
- Many of the implanted memories are so common that it is impossible to rule out subjects remembering experiences that are actually true, or very close to true events.
- Memory contents used in studies range from eating preferences to getting lost in a mall and have little or no similarity to childhood abuse.
- Techniques applied in these studies do not resemble conditions in psychotherapy.

Brewin and Andrews (2016) have proposed three criteria for the evaluation of the quality of autobiographical memory:

1   Autobiographical Belief – A cognitive belief the event did happen.
2   Recollective Experience – A corresponding sensorial complex and complete recollection of the event.
3   Confidence in Memory – Confidence in the truthfulness of the memory.

These three criteria are hard to differentiate and can occur in various combinations. One study showed two-thirds of the subjects believed they remembered seeing TV coverage of an assassination of a Dutch politician. When probing more deeply it turned out that 80% only had an autobiographical belief but no recollective experience (Smeets et al., 2009). Study subjects can believe their memory but have no recollective experience. Study subjects can have a recollective experience of the event, but still have no confidence in the memory. Brewin and Andrews (2016) come to the conclusion:

> While autobiographical belief is a component of memory, we suggest that a 'full' memory for an event, whether true or false, should ideally rest on the combination of the second and third elements. We refer to recollective experiences that have not been demonstrated to be held with confidence as 'partial' memories.

Some might find this pedantic and unnecessary, but the following example should help to illustrate why this kind of detailed evaluation is indeed important.

Shaw and Porter's rich-false-memories study

Shaw and Porter (2015) tried convincing young adults they committed a crime in their youth and the police got involved. They implemented all three paradigms described above (Imagination Inflation, False Feedback, Memory Implantation). Although there are tried and tested evaluation coding systems,

Shaw and Porter developed their own coding system to evaluate the memories of their study subjects. According to their own statement, their coding system was more conservative than the established systems. According to Shaw and Porter's publication, 70% of the subjects developed rich false memories of the implanted criminal offence.

Wade et al. (2017) have challenged Shaw and Porter's success rate. They replicated the study using various blind raters that coded the memories of the subjects using Shaw and Porter's coding system vs. two established systems. Being blind raters they did not know what Shaw and Porter's (2015) or Wade et al.'s (2017) study tried to examine. Using Shaw and Porter's system these raters came to the same conclusion of 70% rich false memories, but using either of the established systems, only 26–30% of the subjects were classified as having false memories with recollective experiences.

In addition, Wade et al. compared a general definition of memory by asking laymen to evaluate when subjects were talking about real memories, without any of the coding schemes. Wade et al. wanted to find out which coding scheme would mirror general opinion. The estimation of the general population coincided with the established coding systems not with Shaw and Porter's system.

Shaw and Porter state that 70% of their study subjects developed rich false memories, but even if we adjust this to 26–30% we have to take into account the subject's confidence in their memories. Different authors take the view that an increase in confidence does not validate drawing any conclusions about the real autobiographical belief if confidence ratings stay in the bottom half of the scale (Mazzoni et al., 2001; Smeets et al., 2005). On a 1–7 Likert scale subjects of Shaw and Porter's study rated their confidence in the false memory with an average of 2.86 (see Table 5.1). With a confidence interval of [2.37, 3.36] no subject's confidence in the false memory reached the middle of

Table 5.1 Table of results from Shaw and Porter's study: "Constructing Rich False Memories of Committing Crime", p. 296.

Condition and memory type	Anxiety		Confidence		Vividness	
	Mean	95% CI	Mean	95% CI	Mean	95% CI
Criminal condition (n = 21)						
False memory	5.48	[5.09, 5.86]	2.86	[2.37, 3.36]	2.68	[2.19, 3.17]
True memory	4.76	[4.26, 5.27]	5.30	[4.92, 5.67]	4.73	[4.29, 5.17]
Noncriminal condition (n = 23)						
False memory	4.52	[3.96, 5.08]	2.76	[2.27, 3.24]	2.59	[2.11, 3.07]
True memory	5.30	[4.92, 5.68]	5.24	[4.80, 5.67]	4.66	[4.18, 5.13]

the scale. According to Brewin and Andrews (2016), we can only speak of partial memories in this situation instead of the "rich false memories" Shaw and Porter propose.

Interestingly, the same effect shows in the "vividness" scale, and only the "anxiety" scale shows a significant mean average of 5.48. In conclusion false memories, while participants report them, do not feel as vivid, do not elicit high confidence, but do elicit higher anxiety than true memories.

Similar results can be found with regard to other sensory components Shaw and Porter enquired about. Only the visual component of false memories in the criminal condition was comfortably above the middle of the scale (see Table 5.2).

It is equally important to take a closer look at the techniques used in false memory research for ethical reasons, as they turn out to be quite questionable. Gaslighting is the name of a play from 1938, which was made into a movie with Ingrid Bergmann in 1944. In the gaslighting story a husband drives his wife insane by manipulating her perceptions and denying her reality. Gaslighting is

> a form of psychological abuse in which false information is presented with the intent of making a victim doubt his or her own memory, perception and sanity. It may simply be the denial by an abuser that previous abusive incidents ever occurred, or it could be the staging of bizarre events by the abuser with the intention of disorienting the victim.
>
> (MacDonald, 2012)

Table 5.2 Table of results from Shaw and Porter's study: "Constructing Rich False Memories of Committing Crime", p. 297

Condition and memory type	Visual		Auditory		Olfactory		Tactile	
	Mean	95% CI	Mean	95% CI	Mean	95% CI	Mean	95% CI
Criminal condition (n = 21)								
False memory	0.86	[0.74, 0.99]	0.39	[0.21, 0.56]	0.14	[0.01, 0.26]	0.30	[0.13, 0.46]
True memory	0.95	[0.88, 1.03]	0.48	[0.30, 0.66]	0.23	[0.08, 0.38]	0.48	[0.30, 0.66]
Noncriminal condition (n = 23)								
False memory	0.85	[0.72, 0.97]	0.41	[0.23, 0.58]	0.15	[0.02, 0.27]	0.29	[0.13, 0.45]
True memory	0.94	[0.85, 1.02]	0.50	[0.32, 0.68]	0.24	[0.09, 0.39]	0.48	[0.30, 0.65]

Different criteria play a significant role in gaslighting:

1   Relationship (1)
Perpetrator and victim have some form of relationship

2   Distortion of reality (2)
The perpetrator aims to distort the victims' reality

3   Irrefutability (3)
The victim has no chance to refute these distortions

4   Adjustment pressure (4)
The perpetrator puts pressure on the victim to agree to his representation of reality

Following are the strategies that were explicitly applied in all of the interviews Shaw and Porter (Shaw & Porter, 2015, p. 294) conducted in their study, and how they relate to gaslighting criteria:

- Building rapport (e.g. asking "How has your semester been?" when they entered the lab)
  - Relationship (1)
- Using facilitators (nodding, smiling, commendation)
  - Relationship (1)
- Purposeful use of pauses and silences (longer pauses often seemed to result in participants providing additional details to cut the silence)
  - Adjustment pressure (4)
- Open-ended prompts ("What else?")
  - Adjustment pressure (4)
- Irrefutable false evidence ("We know from your parents")
  - Irrefutability (3), Distortion of reality (2)
- Social pressure ("Most people are able to retrieve lost memories if they try hard enough")
  - Adjustment pressure (4)
- Suggestive techniques (scripted guided imagery)
  - Depending on how it is conducted: Adjustment pressure (4)

- Presumed additional knowledge ("this sounds like what your parents descri-bed". "I can't give you more details because they have to come from you")

  – Irrefutability (3), Adjustment pressure (4)

- When participants reported that they could not recall the false memory, Shaw responded with disappointment but sympathy ("That's ok. Many people can't recall certain events at first because they haven't thought about them for such a long time".)

  – Relationship (1), Adjustment pressure (4)

- All interviews were conducted in a false office, that openly contained many books on memory and memory retrieval

  – Distortion of reality (2)

This kind of research consciously and deliberately uses techniques that are known to be emotionally abusive, creating emotional strain for their sub-jects – for what reasons?

Some of the memory researchers openly claim their efforts are aimed at preventing innocent convictions, Loftus has said: "It's better to let 10 people who are guilty go than to convict one innocent person" (3sat, 2017). Timothy Hennis was found guilty of raping a woman and then murdering her and her two children. Loftus testified for the defence as an expert witness in Hennis' appeal in 1989 and Hennis was acquitted. In 1989 there were no standard DNA tests. In 2010 Hennis was found guilty before a military court because of positive DNA identification (Fisher, 2016).

It remains curious why researchers like Loftus, Shaw and others conduct their research of false memories with such vehemence. They present their results with apparent triumph and pride in their powers of manipulation. With regards to psychotherapy, it would be entirely reasonable to con-structively research recommendations for good therapy practice. This would enable memory retrieval and processing of unwanted and painful memories, while ensuring our patients do not start to confabulate, and are able to feel trust in their own memories.

Imagination inflation using guided imagery might be the technique from false memory research that closest resembles trauma therapy. Research shows that subjects from studies using imagination inflation rated their false memory as more probable over the course of the studies, but it also shows that only a min-ority of subjects showed these effects, and they were not sustainable. One pro-posal is that this effect only shows the subjects reduced their belief an event did not happen, rather than increasing their belief it did happen (Mazzoni et al., 2001; Smeets et al., 2005). In general, of the three criteria, imagination inflation mainly influences autobiographical belief. But data and statistics of existing stu-dies are hard to compare and evaluate due to varying forms of operationalisation (Brewin & Andrews, 2016).

Conclusions

> The mall study results suggest that if a psychotherapist were to devise a plausible false memory of childhood trauma and tell a client, "I was given this information by your relative who was present at the time", then the client may accept this false account as fully or partially true.
>
> (Crook & Dean, 1999)

On deeper exploration of the research on implanted false memories it becomes clear how complex this issue is, and how misleading the laboratory research results. Independent of our personal opinion, it is our duty as scientists to consider our results critically and to offer them to the public with prudence and caution. Loftus and Shaw present their research results in a simplistic way and do not emphasise enough the caution needed in extrapolating these results into real-life situations. They fail to point out possible limitations (e.g. the absence of confidence) and do not correct mistaken representations by the media: "Although researchers are not responsible for media inaccuracies regarding their research, they are ethically required to attempt to correct inaccuracies to the extent that this is possible" (Crook & Dean, 1999).

Obviously, scientists are not objective cold calculators, but instead are influenced by their personal history just like everyone else. Julia Shaw has said: "Research is me-search ..." (3sat, 2017). Personal (traumatic) histories might indeed have played a role in how some researchers came to be interested in the issue of false memories as well as in the kind of scientific attitude they developed. For instance, Loftus describes how she was sexually abused by a babysitter when she was 6 years old. This memory: "flew out at [her], out of the darkness of the past, hitting [her] with full force" (Loftus & Ketcham, 1991). Shaw reports her father had been mentally ill (Kippenberger & Rosen, 2016), and her autobiographical memory is "not especially good" (3sat, 2017).

In addition to the difficulty in classifying false memories correctly, it is also important to point out the content-related relevance. Most of what is used to be implanted as a false memory in scientific studies nowhere near resembles childhood abuse. Laboratory models are generally less stressful emotionally, and free of the kind of betrayal trauma Freyd (1996) has emphasised, and thus less likely to produce dissociation and forgetting (Freyd, 1993, 1996; DePrince et al. 2012).

For example, one important point of criticism regarding Loftus's "Lost in the Mall" study (Loftus & Pickrell, 1995) relates to the plausibility of the false memory. Being lost in a mall is a common experience and research has shown this kind of plausibility increases autobiographical belief (Brewin & Andrews, 2016). In a study by Pezdeck, Finger and Hodge (1997), the authors tried to implant a more complex false memory, more similar to childhood abuse: The memory of getting painful rectal enemas as a child. This study showed a success rate of 0%. But 15% of the same subjects were led to believe they had been lost in a mall.

When we attempt to draw conclusions about psychotherapy from laboratory research, for example, that psychotherapists could be able to implant false memories of childhood abuse in patients, then we have to focus on the actual comparability of the research with the psychotherapeutic setting. Some scientists researching false memories have used techniques that would never be employed in any ethically acceptable psychotherapy. Above all, no psychotherapist would tell her patients she knows, corroborated by their relatives they were traumatised in childhood. If we look at the psychotherapeutic setting very critically, we might find situations in which the psychotherapist tells their patients that their symptoms are similar to those seen in sexual abuse. Coupling the expert authority of the therapist with the more intense relationship, compared to what we find in short-lived scientific studies, we might assume this could foster confabulation. Whether this would really lead to false memories is questionable. Most of all because real patients in real psychotherapies usually do not like to remember split-off forgotten traumatic experiences as they come with feelings and sensations that are extremely hard to bear, irrevocably overthrowing their conception of their world. Also, psychotherapists do not usually push their patients towards remembering buried childhood abuse and they do not respond with rewarding happiness if they do. In Shaw and Porter's study, Julia Shaw conducted all interviews herself and was motivating subjects to create a "remembering" of the false event. It is very difficult to find research that studies the quality of memory in traumatised psychotherapy patients. It could be interesting to compare the memory-confidence of study subjects in their false memories with the memory-confidence of psychotherapy patients in their recovered memories.

Another issue that hinders the evaluation of false memory research is that many of the scenarios, used as a false memory, are generally so common that we cannot exclude subjects remembering real events or events very similar. Scientists try to circumvent this confounding variable by having relatives confirm study subjects never experienced the event, e.g. getting lost in a mall. However, in addition to empirical clinical experiences we already have research that found statements from relatives to be unreliable (Desjardins & Scoboria, 2007; Porter et al., 1999; Sandberg et al., 1993). Real-life experiences of similar scenario are another problem. Say, one of the subjects has the real experience of being left alone at home at the age of three, and realising this with great fright and despair – this person will be able to fill a false memory of being lost in a mall more easily and vividly because she knows the inherent emotional state. Of course, this kind of blending is something that we as psychotherapists should also be aware of. But it is not improbable that in these cases autobiographical belief with recollection will not lead to sufficient confidence just as we find it in the false memory research. At this point it is important to remember that we as psychotherapists are not the police or detectives nor lawyers. It is not our task to sort through the details of our patient's memories to make them suitable for use in court. Usually patients learn to sort their memories qualitatively. Vogt (2019) introduced a practical approach in differentiating between atmospheric, symbolic and factual memories. An approach that can be a very helpful tool for our patient's self-assessment.

Widespread statements from scientists and popular media emphasise time and again how easy it is to implant false memories: "Moreover, wholly false memories are more common than previously thought, especially for childhood events and, even more alarmingly, it turns out to be almost trivially easy to create false memories in others …" (Conway, 2013, p. 567).

In fact, thorough analysis of the research shows the opposite quite clearly: It is not easy to implant false memories of childhood abuse. Autobiographically believed false memories with recollection and high confidence are rare to non-existent.

References

3sat. (30 March2017). Das getäuschte Gedächtnis [The Deceived Brain] [Video] [retrieved 2 November 2020]. http://www.3sat.de/mediathek/?mode=play&obj=61427.

Brewin, C. R. & Andrews, B. (2016). Creating memories for false autobiographical events in childhood: A systematic review. *Applied Cognitive Psychology.* doi:10.1002/acp.3220

Conway, M. A. (2013). On being a memory expert witness: Three cases. *Memory,* 21, 566–575.

Crook, L. S. & Dean, M. C. (1999). "'Lost in a Shopping Mall' – A Breach of Professional Ethics". *Ethics & Behavior,* 9 (1), 39–50.

DePrince, A. P., Brown, L. S., Cheit, R. E., Freyd, J. J., Gold, S. N., Pezdek, K. & Quina, K. (2012). Motivated Forgetting and Misremembering: Perspectives From Betrayal Trauma Theory. In R.F. Belli (Ed.), *True and False Recovered Memories: Toward a Reconciliation of the Debate (Nebraska Symposium on Motivation 58).* New York: Springer, pp. 193–243.

Desjardins, T. & Scoboria, A. (2007). "You and Your Best Friend Suzy Put Slime in Ms. Smollett's Desk": Producing False Memories with Self-Relevant Details. *Psychonomic Bulletin & Review,* 14, 1090–1095.

Fisher, J. (2 December2016). The Timothy Hennis Triple-Murder Case [retrieved 2 November 2020]. http://jimfishertruecrime.blogspot.de/2014/09/timothy-hennis-search-for-clues-and.html.

Freyd, J. J. (7 August1993). *Controversies around Recovered Memories of Incest and Ritual Abuse.* Presentation at The Center for Mental Health at Foote Hospital's Continuing Education Conference, Ann Arbor, Michigan.

Freyd, J. J. (1996). *Betrayal Trauma: The Logic of Forgetting Childhood Abuse.* Cambridge, MA: Harvard University Press.

Kippenberger, S. & Rosen, B. (10 October2016). Ich misstraue meinen eigenen Erinnerungen [I Distrust My Own Memories] [retrieved 2 November 2020]. http://www.tagesspiegel.de/weltspiegel/sonntag/gedaechtnisforschung-wir-confabulieren-alle/14658386-2.html.

Loftus, E. F. & Ketcham, K. (1991). *Witness for the Defense: The Accused, The Eyewitness, and the Expert Who Puts Memory on Trial.* New York: St. Martin's Press.

Loftus, E. F. & Pickrell, J. E. (1995). The Formation of False Memories. *Psychiatric Annals,* 25 (12), 720–725.

MacDonald, A. (7 November2012). Gaslighting: What It Isn't [retrieved 2 November 2020]. https://alfredmacdonald.com/2012/11/07/gaslighting-what-it-isnt/.

Mazzoni, G. A. L., Loftus, E. F. & Kirsch, I. (2001). Changing Beliefs About Implausible Autobiographical Events: A Little Plausibility Goes a Long Way. *Journal of Experimental Psychology: Applied*, 7, 51–59.

Pezdek, K., Finger, K. & Hodge, D. (1997). Planting False Childhood Memories: The Role Of Event Plausibility. *Psychological Science*, 8 (6), 437–441.

Porter, S., Yuille, J. C. & Lehman, D. R. (1999). The Nature of Real, Implanted, and Fabricated Memories for Emotional Childhood Events: Implications for the Recovered Memory Debate. *Law and Human Behavior*, 23, 517–537.

Sandberg, S., Rutter, M., Giles, S., Owen, A., Champion, L., Nicholls, J. ... & Drinnan, D. (1993). Assessment of Psychosocial Experiences in Child-Hood – Methodological Issues and Some Illustrative Findings. *Journal of Child Psychology and Psychiatry*, 34, 879–897.

Shaw, J. & Porter, S. (2015). Constructing Rich False Memories of Committing Crime. *Psychological Science*, 26 (3), 291–301.

Smeets, T., Merckelbach, H., Horselenberg, R. & Jelicic, M. (2005). Trying to Recollect Past Events: Confidence, Beliefs, and Memories. *Clinical Psychology Review*, 25, 917–934.

Smeets, T., Telgen, S., Ost, J., Jelicic, M. & Merckelbach, H. (2009). What's Behind Crashing Memories? Plausibility, Belief and Memory in Reports of Having Seen Non-Existent Images. *Applied Cognitive Psychology*, 23, 1333–1341.

Vogt, R. (Ed.) (2019). The Traumatised Memory–Protection and Resistance: How traumatic Stress Encrypts Itself in the Body, Behaviour and Soul and How to Detect it. Berlin: Lehmanns Media.

Wade, K. A., Garry, M. & Pezdek, K. (2017). De-Constructing Rich False Memories of Committing Crime: Commentary On Shaw And Porter (2015). *Psychological Science*, 29 (3), 471–476.

Chapter 6

The abuse of science to silence the abused

Ashley Conway

In this chapter Ashley reviews his contribution to Memory in Dispute from 22 years ago. He describes what he considers remains true and where he was wrong – particularly in originally assuming that the problems were due to "experts" who could not see, compared to his realisation now that the problem lies with those who will not see.

I wrote "Shooting the Messenger" more than 20 years ago (Conway, 1998).

Since that time I have continued to work with people who have been traumatised in very diverse ways – ranging from road traffic accidents, military veterans, victims of kidnap, violent assault, terrorist attacks, adults abused in childhood and many more. During this time, I have come across numerous examples of clients where recall of the trauma has been incomplete. In each of these cases I can see no reason why the client might have had any motivation to deliberately mislead.

Here are a few cases that have been associated with memory difficulties:

I worked with a man who was an employee in a bank where there had been an armed robbery. My client had had a shotgun held inches from his face while the robbery took place. When interviewed by the police, he was asked to describe the man who held the gun. To his embarrassment he was unable to do so. The police asked, "Well, was it a black man or white man?" He replied that he didn't know. He could only remember seeing the end of a shotgun barrel very close to his face.

A woman grew up with a physically abusive father. She remembers her father severely beating the family dog in front of her and her older sister, and never seeing the dog again. She said that her memory stops at a certain point in the beating (her father picking up a brick). She reported that her older sister had exactly the same memory, which also stopped at the same point. Two children witnessing the same event, and both memories stopping at the same point. Was the next part of what happened bearable to recall?

A man who was very seriously injured in a terrorist explosion, but did not lose consciousness. He had fragmentary memories of what happened immediately following the explosion. He suffered a very specific flashback to a particular scene, and wanted to know for certain that his memory was right. He spent many months contacting news agencies for footage of the incident. He eventually

DOI: 10.4324/9781003193159-7

found what he wanted: a few seconds of film in which he appeared, showing exactly what his flashback suggested. An image in his head that he found himself almost unable to believe turned out to be completely accurate.

Hearing accounts from people who have been traumatised, and who have fragmented memories of these events is nothing surprising for me, or in my experience police officers who interview the traumatised. Yet, when it comes to experiences of childhood sexual abuse (CSA) the theme of memory of the trauma becomes controversial. Why?

I am going to comment on my 1998 chapter (reprinted below in italics with some minor omissions), and identify how my position has developed since that time.

This brief chapter is a personal perspective, an attempt to identify and examine the allegations of the proponents of the concept of a false memory syndrome. It is not intended as a general review of the field. Questions about the reliability of children's reports and suggestibility of children, which form an important and distinct field, are not addressed here. Instead, the focus is on the issues relating to adults apparently recovering the memory of episodes of childhood sexual abuse, after a period of complete or partial amnesia. Individuals have reported recovering such memories both within and without a therapeutic setting.

Examined here are a number of assumptions, explicit or implicit, that have been derived from material provided by the American and British false memory syndrome movements, the press, and other media and through various personal communications to the author. The assumptions may be summarised as follows:

1   One person can have pseudo-memories implanted by another person.

This is true. Memory is unreliable, and it is the case that people can have mistaken memories implanted or enhanced by another. However, there is a logical flaw that occurs repeatedly in the false memory syndrome message – because some people under some circumstances can have some memories implanted, there is an implicit assumption that where individuals and their alleged abusers disagree over "the truth", then the accuser's memory must be false.

Now, I would ask why there is so little widely-known laboratory research looking at the other side of that coin. Whether false negative memories can be created as well as false positive, i.e. whether somebody can be persuaded that something did not happen, when actually it did. Such research might help to inform us more about failure to recall. This avoidance of looking at false negative memories maintains a bias in this research. Twenty years on, my perception of this is not complicated. The false memory syndrome (FMS) advocates do not want evidence of false negatives – that we can experience something and then be persuaded that it did not happen, because that would not suit their narrative.

2   Because they are gullible, deluded, have axes to grind, or are greedy, therapists persuade clients to have false beliefs of having been sexually abused in childhood.

There is no evidence that anyone has ever had a false belief implanted that they were sexually abused as a child. Such evidence is not possible to acquire, as it is not possible to know for sure that a person has not been sexually abused, and it would not be ethical to conduct research attempting to implant such a belief. It may be the case that some therapists are gullible or hold incorrect beliefs. Yapko's much-quoted data (e.g. Yapko, 1994) shows that, of his surveyed therapists, 47% believed that hypnosis improved reliability of recall, 54% believed that patients could recall events as far back as birth, and 28% believed that hypnosis could be used to recover memories of past lives. The first of these beliefs is a factual error, the second and third have little or no scientific evidence to support them. The false memory lobby implication is that if therapists believe these things, then they will believe in anything.

Some therapists may have axes to grind – some do have a particular belief that childhood sexual abuse lies at the heart of many adult problems, and this preconception may indeed bias their approach. Of course, it is also the case that many therapists and academics have preconceptions that child abuse is over-stated, and that this creates in them a bias of denial of adults' reports of abuse. This is a frequent complaint of those trying to tell someone about their memories of abuse. Both child abuse specialists and false memory groups may contain individuals who have their own causes to advance. The false memory groups derive much of their energy (and presumably funds) from people accused of child abuse – so any difficulty that they might have in maintaining neutrality is, perhaps, unsurprising.

The final part of this assumption is that therapists stand to make themselves richer by persuading their clients that they have childhood abuse in their background and need prolonged and expensive therapy. My own experience, and that of colleagues to whom I have spoken, is that child abuse is actually not a good field to pursue if money is the main motivation. Victims of extreme childhood abuse are often dysfunctional, which is frequently associated with financial hardship. In the United Kingdom at least, the situation seems to me to be the opposite of that which is alleged, and that in fact therapists fre-quently give a great deal of time and energy to working with people who have been abused for little reward or no payment at all.

As I pointed out 20 years ago, and I feel even more strongly about this now, bias about beliefs in reports of abuse still frequently occur in the opposite direc-tion – there are groups of people who seem to have a fixation on avoiding the evidence and denying the reality of the incidence of child sexual abuse.

The other point in this section was whether therapists make significant financial gain from creating a belief in CSA. In reality, working clinically with survivors of CSA is not a smart way to get rich – survivors are not usually a good source of income.

However, according to Newberry (2020), Professor Elizabeth Loftus has appeared as an expert witness in more than 300 trials, and charges around $500 an hour for her legal work. She reports that critics say that Loftus's pattern of testifying for alleged offenders and not their accusers, shows an inherent bias. And adds "prosecutors tend to have tighter budgets than wealthy defendants". So, far from the claims of therapists getting rich in this arena, working as a witness for the defence appears a much more lucrative option. In fact, "It is almost as if the field has been driven more by the needs of legal defence teams than by true scientific enquiry" (McMaugh & Middleton, 2020).

3   Hypnosis makes inaccuracies more likely and increases confidence in these inaccuracies.

> *It is sometimes true that hypnosis can be used to increase confidence in inaccurate memories. But it is also true that there is considerable evidence that hypnosis can also enhance accurate recall (e.g. Ewin, 1994; Nemiah, 1985). Again, the other side of the story is omitted by the false memory syndrome advocates. It would seem sensible to suggest that nothing about the truth or falsehood of hypnotically recovered memory can be assumed without corroborating evidence.*

Hypnosis can help induce a state of relative calm where clients can work through their traumatic experiences without being overwhelmed by them. Good clinical research, with carefully applied use of hypnosis, by trained clinicians, might reveal whether hypnosis has a positive role to play in recall and healing from trauma. The original American False Memory Syndrome Foundation advisory board included at least two experts on hypnosis: Martin Orne and Ernest Hilgard. I wonder why they did not promote such research?

4   A number of accusers have retracted; therefore, accusations are unreliable.

> *It is true that accusers have retracted, but this does not mean that accusations are unreliable. In its statement on memories of sexual abuse, the American Psychiatric Association (APA, 1993) reports that retracting can follow an initial report of childhood abuse in victims with documented abuse. One of the few studies on retracting suggests that this is frequently part of the disclosure process, and the retraction is often subsequently withdrawn and the accusation maintained (Gonzalez, Water man, Kelly, McCord & Oliveri, 1993).*

Retraction, as I pointed out then, is a complex issue, and may be a part of the disclosure process for some, with the retraction being subsequently withdrawn. Oversimplifying this complex area leads to greater confusion and less understanding.

5   Having an explanation for one's problems by claiming child sexual abuse is an easy cop-out for the accusers – it means that they can blame someone else for their problems.

The suggestion that alleging child abuse is an easy option has no foundation in reality – it is simply untrue. Coming to terms with childhood abuse is a long and painful process. On the other hand, it could be argued that denial is a much more comfortable (but perhaps ultimately less sane) option both for victims and for their families.

My original thoughts about an abuse explanation being a cop-out are unchanged. Denial is a much less stressful route than reporting abuse.

6   There is no such thing as traumatic amnesia, repression, and therefore recovered memory, and greater levels of trauma are more likely to be remembered.

It is clearly untrue that there is no such thing as traumatic amnesia. Inability to recall important aspects of a trauma is a diagnostic criterion for post-traumatic stress disorder and dissociative amnesia (APA: DSM-V, 2013). The issues of repression and recovered memory have been addressed in a number of studies. Herman and Schatzow (1987) studied 53 patients in childhood abuse survivor groups; 64% reported at least some degree of amnesia, and 9 out of 12 of the most violently abused women had experienced prolonged amnesia. Briere and Conte (1989) studied 468 subjects with self-reported childhood abuse histories; 60% reported amnesic episodes, with greater violence and death threats being associated with greater likelihood of amnesia. Cameron (1994) reported a study surveying 72 women in therapy to deal with the long-term effects of childhood abuse; she reported that "It was harder to find research participants who had always remembered their abuse than ones who had been at least partially amnesic to it". These studies involved subjects who were self-diagnosed and whose accounts were retrospective. Berliner and Williams (1994) cited a study by Widom and Morris involving a longitudinal follow up of documented child abuse cases, which found a substantial proportion of the sample failing to recall the sexual abuse experience. A major prospective study has been reported by Williams (1994a), in which 129 female abuse victims were followed up an average of seventeen years after documented abuse. 38% did not recall the abusive event, and those who were assaulted by someone they knew were more likely to be amnesic. The evidence from these studies could be interpreted as providing empirical support for the existence of traumatic amnesia, repression, and recovered memory. It also specifically contradicts the assumption that greater trauma is more likely to be remembered, actually finding the opposite to be the case.

This sixth point is the one that I would pick out now as perhaps the most important. One of the biggest changes in my awareness of the field in recent years has been seeing how data derived from experimental research, often with students, has been inappropriately and misleadingly assumed to inform us about memory processes involved in the recall of abuse during childhood. Referring to some of these FMS research projects, McMaugh and Middleton (2020) state, "There is nothing that happens in therapy, nor in a legal investigation, that is anything like bringing in a trusted family member to lie to clients, along with possibly supplying some doctored photos!"

Since the 1990s it has become clearer that trauma has a significant impact on memory. Neuroscience advances have shown us that brain activity can be grossly disrupted by trauma. Memory processes during and after traumatic experiences are unlike memory processing during non-traumatic times. Van der Kolk (2014) is an excellent source on the development of this new understanding: "The imprints of traumatic experiences are organised not as coherent logical narratives but in fragmented sensory and emotional traces: images, sounds and physical sensations (p. 176)". And "when people fully recall their traumas, they 'have' the experience. They are engulfed by the sensory or emotional elements of the past" (p. 219).

Traumatic memories are fundamentally different from other kinds of memory from the past; they are dissociated. That is, there is a disruption of the normal integration of consciousness, memory, emotion, perception and behaviour. As van der Kolk says: "Dissociation is the essence of trauma" (p. 66). Dissociative symptoms can potentially disrupt every area of psychological functioning. He also points out that childhood trauma is radically different from traumatic stress in adults, and that different forms of abuse have different impacts on various brain areas at different stages of development (p. 140).

Dissociative identity disorder (DID) is the most severe of all dissociative disorders, and its features include recurrent amnesia. Recent research (Reinders et al., 2019) has demonstrated that individuals with DID can be distinguished from healthy controls on the basis of abnormal brain morphology. In this study individuals with DID also scored significantly higher than control subjects for traumatic experiences on five adverse life event categories: emotional neglect, emotional abuse, physical abuse, sexual abuse and sexual harassment.

With regard to recall of abusive childhood experiences:

> There have in fact been hundreds of scientific publications spanning well over a century documenting how the memory of trauma can be repressed, only to resurface years or decades later … Total memory loss is most common in childhood sexual abuse, with incidence ranging from 19 percent to 38%.

And "Every single scientific study of memory of childhood sexual abuse, whether prospective or retrospective, whether studying clinical samples or general population samples, finds that a certain percentage of sexually abused individuals forget, and later remember, their abuse" (Van der Kolk, 2014, note on p. 398 re. p. 190). And Ross Cheit (2015) has provided us with a remarkable online resource of over 100 corroborated cases of recovered memory.

At the time of writing the British False Memory Society, supported by its scientific advisors, states on its website (bfms.org.uk) "sexual abuse is easy to remember and extremely difficult to forget. Genuine victims unfortunately cannot repress or forget what has happened to them". But, as noted above, the inability to remember an important aspect of a traumatic event, typically due to dissociative amnesia, has long been a diagnostic criterion for post-traumatic stress disorder. Is the suggestion from the advisory board of the BFMS that trauma experts have got this wrong for decades? Or that sexual abuse is not traumatic? And is the implication of the BFMS statement that those who have experienced traumatic amnesia are not "genuine victims"? These are all extreme minority opinions that appear to be presented as facts. As McMaugh and Middleton (2020) state, "the 'false memory' movement enabled society to ignore a whole new generation of abused children".

In reality "it is possible, temporarily, to entirely forget an experience of child sexual abuse or aspects of the abuse. Dissociation and complete forgetting were significant among a sample of victims whose age at the onset of abuse was in early childhood" (Goodman-Delahunty et al., 2017, p. 89). And "Dozens of studies have demonstrated that children who are extensively abused prior to adolescence frequently exhibit either partial or complete amnesia for the abusive events ... Many studies have demonstrated evidence that it is common to forget, and later remember, parts or all of the serious traumatic events such as child sexual abuse" (Stavropoulos & Kezelman, 2018, p. 22).

Freyd and Birrell (2013, p. 126) clarify that disclosure of traumatic memories is highly dependent on the safety of the context in which disclosure is received and responded to.

Both Goodman-Delahunty et al. (2017) and Stavropoulos & Kezelman (2018) also report that studies show that corroboration rates for discontinuous, unreported traumatic memories are similar to those for continuous memories. Stavropoulos and Kezelman (2018) state:

> it is critical to be aware that contrary to the implied and overt claims of many 'false memory' proponents, research upholds that recovered memories are no less likely to be reliable than explicit consciously recalled memories which were never forgotten in the first place.
>
> (p. 33)

The World Health Organisation's International Classification of Diseases (ICD-11) is planned to include a new diagnosis of complex post-traumatic stress disorder (CPTSD; Karatzias et al., 2017). Childhood, multiple and interpersonal trauma and sexual violence are all most likely associated with CPTSD as opposed to PTSD in both clinical and population samples. Karatzias et al. (2017) make reference to "traumatised individuals who possess no clear memory of their index trauma ... possibly due to childhood traumatization ..."

My conclusion now is that contrived laboratory studies with students, trying to induce a false memory of a relatively plausible event, have little or nothing to inform us about the processes of memory and recall of childhood trauma – and to suggest otherwise is simply misleading.

> *The demands of the position of the false memory syndrome groups are tricky: we are asked to believe that memory is unreliable, but in only one direction – that we can have false positive memories (we can be led to believe that something did happen, when in fact it did not), but not false negatives (we cannot apparently be amnesic about something that did happen), and that false memories can be implanted in adults by persuasive therapists, but not, apparently, in children by persuasive adults (see, e.g.* Marsden, 1994). *Additionally, a claim of abuse is considered incredible, whereas a retraction by the same person is credible. When individuals re-accuse, do they become incredible again?*
>
> *Both the American Psychiatric Association (* APA, 1993) *and the British Psychological Society (Morton et al., 1995) statements on recovered memories acknowledge the possibility of dissociative amnesia.*

In good science data is gathered and a theory is formed. In bad science a theory is formed and the evidence is gathered to fit the theory. Now, after 20 years, I think that my 1998 chapter was naive. I thought that there was a debate about matters of fact, of science. Now, I do not think that the conflict has much to do with fact or science. I think that the problem is to do with the dogma of those who aim to deny the incidence and consequences of CSA.

Merchants of Doubt (Oreskes & Conway, 2010) is an informative book written to describe how vested interests have manipulated the media, to mislead and confuse in areas of great importance to society, including smoking, acid rain and climate change. From their account, I have derived a list of strategies used by those with vested interests to mislead the world away from the real science: they create an institute, with scientific advisors who can use their credentials to present themselves as authorities. The advisors cherry-pick data to advance a position, present ideas as if they were facts and use their authority to try to discredit any science they do not like. They use the mass media, making simplified, dramatic statements to capture public attention and draw in journalists to give their minority views more credence than they deserve. They then use these press stories, quoting them as if they were facts. If there is an individual whose opinions are contradictory to the desired line, *ad hominem* attacks are an option.

To a neutral observer it might well appear that the false memory protagonists have closely followed this template.

The FMS lobby have promoted the idea that there are "Memory Wars" – a battle between naive therapists and the wise false memory scientists. The UK and the US FMS organisations were initially set up by the accused to defend the interests of the accused. But they talk as if they are some neutral guardians of the truth. They deny the reality of the phenomena of dissociation and traumatic amnesia, and this is simply bad science. As well as the victim of abuse, they have added another source to blame – the therapist for helping give the abused a voice. But in reality "only a very small percentage of people recover memories of child sexual abuse in therapy" (Goodman-Delahunty et al., 2017, p. 144).

How does such a small group come to have such a powerful voice? As described by Oreskes and Conway – there is a clever use of the national media. In this way a small number of people can have large, negative impacts, especially if they are organised, determined, and have access to power. When the film *Spotlight* came out it highlighted the extent of abuse by priests in Boston, and the way in which those in power covered up the priests' abuse. How would FMS advocate Elizabeth Loftus deal with this? By Tweeting a link to an article telling us "Why Spotlight is a Terrible Film" (Loftus Tweet of 29 February 2016). The first line of the article that we are directed to is: "I don't believe the victims". It goes on to say, "I don't believe the ... lawyers or the *Boston Globe*'s Spotlight team" or "the prosecutors who pursued tainted cases or the therapists who revived junk science or the juries that sided with them or the judges who failed to act justly". So that becomes the explanation for what happened – *everyone* was wrong. A further example of the success in creating confusion and a blind belief in the reality of FMS was illustrated in an article on allegations about Harvey Weinstein's accusers (adult women reporting continual memory of sexual harassment by him) – "I suspect that false memory syndrome has increased the velocity of these tales ..." (Emily Sheffield, fashion editor, and sister-in-law of a former British Prime Minister, in the *London Evening Standard* 12 October 2017).

In an article published in *The Psychologist* one of the Scientific Advisors to the British False Memory Society reports an interest in researching "ostensibly paranormal experiences". He writes: "It is worth emphasising that exactly the same techniques are used to 'recover' memories of alien abduction and past lives as are used to 'recover' allegedly repressed memories of childhood sexual abuse ..." (French, 2018). This is a classic example of casting doubt by association. Linking alien abduction to child sexual abuse is not just insulting to those who have been abused – it creates confusion where there could be clarity. It is unclear why the British Psychological Society continues to enable obfuscation about such a serious issue in its house publication, circulated to tens of thousands of psychologists. The belief that there is no such thing as traumatic amnesia, and that hundreds of thousands of people report child sexual abuse because they have been brain-washed by deluded therapists, is a topic worthy of scientific research by those interest in anomalistic psychology. Hopefully, the real science will prevail in the very near future.

A further example of distracting focus is the use of *ad hominem* attacks. One example is how to deal with a former President of the American Psychological Association when he reported awkward information and opinion. Koocher (2014) described what he considered to be ethically inappropriate behaviour by Elizabeth Loftus, and additionally stated that he had been told that Loftus resigned from the American Psychological Association because she had been tipped off that there had been complaints made to the association about her, enabling her to resign before the ethics investigation could be initiated. So, how did Loftus respond? Simple – tweet that he is dishonest, or in fact that he is a "Slimeball liar" (Loftus, Tweet of 11 October 2015).

In dodging reality, one strategy is to respond to a perceived criticism by portraying yourself as the victim (coincidentally as abusers frequently do – see reference to DARVO below). In her 2013 TED talk, Elizabeth Loftus states: "I became part of a disturbing trend in America where scientists are being sued for simply speaking out on matters of great public controversy". But the litigation issue was not about speaking out on matters of great public controversy. A few moments earlier she reported the real reason that she was being sued: "for defamation and invasion of privacy". Of course, good science involves good ethics. The issue at stake in Loftus's comment arose because she co-authored an article for a newsstand magazine (Loftus & Guyer, 2002a, 2002b) in which she gave many unnecessary clues to the identity of the subject of a case history, in which the subject was assured anonymity. The case history ran in direct opposition to the FMS position, and it would appear that ethics were cast aside to achieve a goal – the erasure of a case history which ran contrary to the FMS storyline.

Once planted, the FMS narratives do not easily go away. Child sex abuse is an enormous problem. And to deal with it we have to address the campaigns of disinformation. To understand the conflict, we should not make the mistake of assuming that this is simply a scientific debate. We have to consider the cultural and the political, and probably the psychological and possible financial factors too. If we do not think more broadly about how issues around CSA affect people (including "experts") and our society, then I do not think that we will understand why memory is in dispute.

> *For a family to be destroyed by a false accusation of abuse is a terrible experience, and every effort should be made to avoid such an event. The false memory syndrome groups may therefore have something important to offer, but polarisation (right/wrong, true/false) of highly complex issues does not help.*
>
> *Academics in this field may be dealing with complex ethical issues, and those who have lent their names to these causes may become discouraged by this lack of rigour. The scare stories and one-sided anecdotes may be swallowed by a willing and gullible press, but if serious debate is to progress amongst academics and clinicians, then a much more scholarly attitude will be needed.*

Sadly, 20 years on, the same stories and one-sided anecdotes are still being swallowed by a gullible press, and sadder still by some mental health professionals.

"False memory" accusations may be used as one of a number of the weapons of DARVO – an acronym for Deny, Attack, and Reverse Victim and Offender (Freyd, 1997), where perpetrators and their supporters use active strategies to confuse and silence their victims and the media.

Now it is acknowledged that "Memory researchers motivated by their own agendas and interests do not necessarily respond to acknowledged research gaps" (Goodman-Delahunty et al., 2017, p. 36) and "Contemporary research findings demonstrate that concerns about the prevalence of false memories of child sexual abuse appear to have been exaggerated" (p. 144).

This message appeared on the FMSF website in January 2020:

> After 27 years, the FMS Foundation dissolved on 31 December 2019. During the past quarter-century, a large body of scientific research and legal opinions on the topics of the accuracy and reliability of memory and recovered memories has been created ... The need for the FMS Foundation diminished dramatically over the years.

What does this actually mean? Well, as summarised above, a large body of evidence has been created that demonstrates very clearly that many of the assertions of the false memory groups are simply untrue. So the need for a society that promotes harmful information is ... zero.

The misleading FMS propaganda endured in the press and in lecture theatres and court rooms for decades. Why? The untrue statement that CSA cannot be forgotten is still on the British FMS website at the time of writing, and this and other deceptions are endorsed by eminent psychologists on the BFMS Scientific Advisory Board. It is hard to imagine that the false memory societies would have gained such traction with the media without this kind of endorsement. Way back in 1993 Pamela Birrell wrote an open letter to the advisory board members of the False Memory Syndrome Foundation (Freyd & Birrell, 2013, pp. 157–61):

> as a clinical psychologist, I have seen the damage done by this organisation to survivors of *documented* sexual abuse as they struggle to establish their own reality and to deal with the overwhelming pain of their trauma ... I am writing this letter to ask all of you to examine your motives and to look at the consequences of your membership on the advisory board of this particular foundation ...

Only two members of the board ever responded to the letter, and their responses were "terse and uncompromising", basically stating that they did not see this side of the controversy at all, and were not willing to engage in dialogue.

Misrepresentation of known psychological evidence is a breach of British Psychological Society ethical guidelines. But when a formal complaint was made to the BPS about the advisors to the British False Memory Society doing just that, the reply was, "We considered the ethical issue here to be one of freedom of expression. In the view of the Committee, the Scientific advisors are free to provide advice in good faith, as either academics and/or professionals to other organisations". So, far from castigating those misleading the world to the detriment of the abused, the BPS has historically turned a blind eye to the gross misrepresentations of psychological knowledge, and in fact granted FMS dogmatists honours, and many column inches in its publications.

As noted above, disclosure of traumatic memories is highly dependent on the safety of the context in which disclosure is received and responded to. The misinformation about false memory that has been fed to the world has frequently made the context of disclosure *un*safe. Thus, a belief in the FMS propaganda is likely to decrease the likelihood of abuse being reported. Was this a conscious intent?

Is the conflict over the real science of traumatic memory over? We need to be rigorous in understanding what has happened, and what drives the need for the denial of a person's history – whether individual, societal, and perhaps particularly from academics and mental health professionals and their representative bodies. We need to learn lessons about misrepresentation of the facts, the abuse of the science and the abuse of the truth – and why that abuse is being acted out and not called out.

Now that the US FMSF seems to have reached its demise, a new way of discounting victims' accounts has already appeared. In acting for Harvey Weinstein's defence team FMS promoter Elizabeth Loftus presented the idea of "the phenomenon known as 'voluntary unwanted sex'". This was defined in court papers as "sex that is undesired, but that the person chooses to engage in" and argued that it is likely to lead to confusion over consent. So people may be consenting and not realising it? Is voluntary unwanted sex (VUS) simply another way to make people feel unsafe about disclosing abuse? Is VUS the new FMS?

In reviewing my 20-year old chapter "Shooting the Messenger", my conclusion is that we are well overdue, switching our attention from the messenger (client or clinician) and should instead turn a spotlight on those doing the shooting.

References

APA. (1993). *Statement on Memories of Sexual Abuse.* Washington, DC: American Psychiatric Association.

APA. (2013). *Diagnostic and Statistical Manual of Mental Disorders 5th Edition (DSM-V).* Washington, DC: American Psychiatric Publishing.

Berliner, L. & Williams, L. M. (1994). Memories of Child Sexual Abuse: A Response To Lindsay and Read. *Applied Cognitive Psychology*, 8, 379–387.

Briere, J. & Conte, J. (1989). *Amnesia in Adults Molested as Children Testing Theories of Repression.* Paper presented at the annual meeting of the American Psychological Association, New Orleans.

Cameron, C. (1994). Veterans of a Secret War-Survivors Of Childhood Sexual Trauma Compared to Vietnam War Veterans With PTSD. *Journal of Interpersonal Violence*, 9, 117–132.

Cheit, R. (2015). http://blogs.brown.edu/recoveredmemory/case-archive/.

Conway, A. (1998). Shooting the Messenger. In V. Sinason (Ed), *Memory in Dispute.* London: Karnac.

Ewin, D. (1994). Many Memories Retrieved With Hypnosis Are Accurate. *American Journal of Clinical Hypnosis*, 36, 174–176.

French, C. (April, 2018). Reaching Brenda from the Chip Shop. *The Psychologist*, 45.

Freyd, J. J. (1997). Violations of Power, Adaptive Blindness, and Betrayal Trauma Theory. *Feminism & Psychology*, 7, 22–32.

Freyd, J. & Birrell, P. (2013). *Blind to Betrayal*. London: John Wiley & Sons.

Gonzalez, L. S., Waterman, J., Kelly, R. J., McCord, J. & Oliveri, M. K. (1993). Children's Patterns of Disclosures And Recantations of Sexual and Ritualistic Abuse Allegations in Psychotherapy. *Child Abuse and Neglect*, 17, 281–289.

Goodman-Delahunty, J., Nolan, M. A. & van Gijn-Grosvenor, E. L. (2017). Empirical Guidance on the Effects of Child Sexual Abuse on Memory and Complainants' Evidence. Sydney, Australia: Royal Commission into Institutional Responses to Child Sexual Abuse.

Herman, J. L. & Schatzow, E. (1987). Recovery and Verification of Memories of Childhood Sexual Trauma. *Psychoanalytic Psychology*, 4, 1–14.

Karatzias, T.*et al.* (2017). PTSD and Complex PTSD: ICD-11 updates on concept and measurement in the UK, USA, Germany and Lithuania. *European Journal of Psychotraumatology*, 8 (7).

Koocher, G. P. (2014) Research Ethics and Private Harms. *Journal of Interpersonal Violence*, 29, 3267–3276.

Loftus, E. (11 October2015).. https://twitter.com/eloftus1.

Loftus, E. (29 February2016).. https://twitter.com/eloftus1.

Loftus, E. F. & Guyer, Melvin J. (2002a). Who Abused Jane Doe? The Hazards of the Single Case Study: Part 1. *Skeptical Inquirer*, 26 (3), 24–32.

Loftus, E. F. & Guyer, Melvin J. (2002b). Who Abused Jane Doe? Part 2. *Skeptical Inquirer*, 26 (4): 37–40, 44.

Loftus, E. (2013). *How Reliable is your Memory?*TED Global talk,June 2013. https://www.ted.com/talks/elizabeth_loftus_the_fiction_of_memory

Marsden, B. (1994). False Memory Syndrome – True or False? *European Journal of Clinical Hypnosis*, 48–55.

McMaugh, K. & Middleton, W. (21 January2020). The Rise and Fall of the False Memory Syndrome Foundation. *ISSTD News*. https://news.isst-d.org/the-rise-and-fall-of-the-false-memory-syndrome-foundation.

Morton, J., Andrews, B., Bekerian, D., Brewin, C., Davies, G. & Mollon, P. (1995). *Recovered Memories: The Report of the Working Party of the British Psychological Society*. Leicester: British Psychological Society.

Newberry, L. (6 February2020) This "False Memory" Expert Has Testified in Hundreds of Trials. Now She's Been Hired by Harvey Weinstein. *Los Angeles Times*. https://www.latimes.com/california/story/2020-02-06/false-memory-expert-testify-harvey-weinstein-trial.

Nemiah, J. C. (1985). Dissociative Disorders (Hysterical Neurosis, Dissociative Type). In: H. I. Kaplan & B. J. Sadock (Eds), *Comprehensive Textbook of Psychiatry* (4th ed.). Baltimore: Williams & Wilkins.

Oreskes, N. & Conway, E. M. (2010). *Merchants of Doubt*. New York: Bloomsbury Press. 2010.

Reinders, A. A. T. S.*et al.* (2019). Aiding the Diagnosis of Dissociative Identity Disorder: Pattern Recognition Study of Brain Biomarkers. *The British Journal of Psychiatry*, 215 (3), 536–544.

Stavropoulos P. A. & Kezelman C. A. (2018) *The Truth of Memory and The Memory of Truth: Different Types of Memory and the Significance for Trauma.* NSW, Australia: Blue Knot Foundation.

Van der Kolk, B. (2014). *The Body Keeps the Score.* New York: Penguin.

Williams, L. M. (1994a). Recall of Childhood Trauma: A Prospective Study of Women's Memories of Child Sexual Abuse. *Journal of Consulting and Clinical Psychology*, 62, 1167–1176.

Yapko, M. D. (1994). Suggestibility and Repressed Memories of Abuse: A Survey of Psychotherapist's Beliefs. *American Journal of Clinical Hypnosis*, 36, 163–171.

Chapter 7

False memory syndrome

Susie Orbach

In this chapter, written nearly 25 years ago at the height of discussion on sexual abuse and its denial in the form of the propagation of false memory syndrome, Susie Orbach shows the part that feminism played in the understanding of the extent of abuse against women and children. She examines the processes of personal denial in the consulting room, as well as societal denial and the role of the media.

In the spring of 1993, I wrote a piece in my *Guardian* column raising concerns about the take-up in the media of the so-called false memory syndrome. I expressed my surprise and concern that so many column inches were being devoted to a discussion of parents claiming to be unjustly accused by their children rather than to what I considered the more serious problem of the sexual violation of children.

I argued that – as Jeffrey Masson (1984), Judith Herman Lewis (Herman, 1981, 1992) and others have argued – psychoanalysis has a complex and reasonably dishonourable history in relation to the acceptance of the veracity of reports of childhood sexual abuse. Since Freud abandoned the seduction theory in the late 1890s and transferred his understanding of the accounts of his patients' childhood memories of sexual encounters with parents to the realm of internal phantasy, psychotherapy and its allied fields have tended to overlook both the existence and the real trauma of sexual abuse.

When women began to claim for themselves the right to speak of their own experience, they could articulate what life was like from their vantage point. They described how work, mothering, relationships, the health system, the education system looked to them, how the interface between the public world and the private world of the family operated, how their intimate relationships functioned or didn't function, how there were pressures on them to be the emotional support system and emotional sewage-treatment plant for everyone. Once these perceptions were given space so that women's subjective experiences could be described and validated, it was possible to create the kind of climate in the general population that meant that women could reveal secrets they had kept about some of the emotional and sexual violence that they had sustained in their childhood.

DOI: 10.4324/9781003193159-8

As women came forward to testify to the brutality that they lived with, it became obvious that childhood sexual abuse was far more widespread than common sense had allowed one to think. Women's recognition of their own history and the valuing of women's lives, which had begun to be on the agenda over the last 20 years, led in turn to a recognition that children's experiences needed to be valued and recognised too, and there was a shift in how we perceived children. Children were no longer simply the possessions of their parents but citizens with rights, including the right to be heard and a right to a childhood free of abuse.

This shift in the way in which children were regarded led to people listening more to children, just as we began to listen more to women. Out of the mouths of young children – both girls and boys – came horrific reports of deeply inappropriate sexual, violent and sadistic relationships foisted on them, and as a society we were required to think about what on earth was going on. It became obvious that many children were surviving in perilous situations and that they were embedded in dangerous and hurtful relationships. Child protection workers and doctors moved in various ways to safeguard the children, and a public conversation about the level of sexual abuse ensued.

This public conversation is marked by a great deal of passion and hysteria. There are many parties to the conversation, although they are not often all heard, and the debate is often characterised by a kind of political fundamentalism – "All men are potential abusers" or "The children just make up what they want the adults to hear". But in truth there are other voices straining to be heard and straining to understand and position themselves *vis-à-vis* these polarities. For many, the idea of sexual abuse is so repellent and so unfathomable that its widescale existence is incomprehensible: to accept that so many have been violated forces a deep reconsideration of human behaviour. It challenges their sense of what it means to be human. For others, a certain kind of abuse can be accepted where another kind is negated. Colleagues of mine, for example, will say, "Yes, I accept sexual abuse but ritual abuse – now, that is just not on. Are you sure you aren't being bamboozled here or getting over-involved?" For others, confusion, fear, and conflicting feelings overwhelm them, and the public discussion with its fundamentalist demands makes it hard for them to talk.

In my *Guardian* column, I wrote that an interesting phenomenon from my perspective as a clinician – as a general psychotherapist rather than someone who works in the area of sexual abuse – is the discomfort and resistance that I observe when my clients or patients encounter in themselves evidence of sexual abuse in their childhood. They tell of it, but then withdraw from the knowledge of what they have said. Unlike children who are in the midst of an abusive situation, adults who appeared to have been abused in childhood, far from rushing off to accuse their parents, were extremely hesitant to acknowledge what might be staring us both in the face. They would do anything to conceal this knowledge from themselves. They would rather not know, not confront their history, not believe.

I speculated that, if the survivors were amnesic, then it was possible that the perpetrators – many of whom had been consistently abused themselves when children – were similarly amnesic or dissociated when they were committing acts of sexual abuse. I did not say this to let them off the hook, but to extend insights from clinical practice with survivors. I return to this issue of secrecy and resistance to the acknowledgement of abuse shortly in more detail. For the moment, I want to take you through my experience and thinking following the publication of my *Guardian* piece.

The piece came out, and I was besieged by correspondence from parents who alleged that they had been accused, falsely, by their children of sexual abuse. My first response was to think that I had seriously underestimated the phenomenon. To be sure, I had acknowledged in the article that it was possible that parents were being falsely accused, but I set this within the context that the main issue was the abuse of children and I questioned whether the focus on false memory was not some kind of backlash both against feminism and a response to our inability as a culture to deal with the horror of child molestation. I also wondered why adult children would be accusing their parents falsely. Like the therapist I am, my thought was that if sexual abuse had not occurred, then something had gone dreadfully wrong for the children to have turned in this manner against their parents. We know that there can be deep conflict between parents and children, but for a child to express that conflict through a false allegation of sexual abuse struck me as indicative of something quite serious.

So the letters arrived, and my assistant Petra Fried and I read them. Some of these letters were extremely moving. All were deeply upsetting because they detailed fractured relationships in which the parents were inexplicably bereft of a relationship with their children. The letters fell into two camps: those that struck one as the absolutely genuine outpourings of broken-hearted parents, and those that disquieted me in a different way. The latter read as wooden – one might almost say they were formulaically composed. Although we did not decipher this in all of the letters in this category, there were certainly some containing slips ("I did abuse my daughter" when the writer intended "I didn't abuse my daughter"), which was extremely interesting, and all included a curious reference to the fact that the writers were not anti-feminist.

I was determined to keep an open mind and to accept that I had seriously underestimated the number of parents falsely accused. I felt that there was incontrovertible evidence that some people trained in hypnotherapy were using suggestion to induce an explanation of sexual abuse for the distress that their patients came to them with. I was prepared to consider that people were more suggestible than perhaps I had realised and that false memory was something to be grappled with.

This was one strain of my thinking, and during the rest of the year I encountered many people who would want to reinforce that line of argument. At the same time, I was concerned to discover how many people in my professional and wider personal world dismissed the relevance of sexual abuse and called those who worried about it zealots or perverts themselves.

But a meeting with Roger Scotford on television has continued to worry me about the British False Memory Society and its influence in generating articles like the Simon Hoggart piece in *The Observer* of 23 March 1994, which argued that rational argument is impossible (Hoggart, 2004). Hoggart has likened the pressure on parents falsely accused to the "Red Scare" that swept North America in the 1950s. Such articles promote the idea that the sexual abuse of children is secondary to the major problem of false memory.

I left the BBC studio feeling very uneasy about some of the membership of his organisation, and I was alarmed to see academics and psychoanalysts joining his advisory board. It did not seem parallel to parents and academics who join organisations such as SANE or MENCAP.

Since then, Valerie Sinason's brave and deeply disturbing collection *Treating Survivors of Satanist Abuse* (Sinason, 1994) has been published, and we have seen a new round of denial and dismissal that such things can happen. BBC2's Newsnight, in trying to deal with the question of child abuse, promised those they wished to interview (the agencies and individuals involved with the aftercare of survivors) a non-biased programme. The result was far from that – it was as partisan as one could possibly go in the direction of proclaiming false memory to be the fundamental problem, not sexual abuse.

Those who work in child protection and with those who have been abused must suffer appalling feelings of outrage and helplessness as they see mendaciously mischaracterised as fantasy what we know to be happening. It is as though what had to be kept secret, what had to be denied, what could not be spoken of by the children was now being done on a public level. The truth of sexual abuse had pierced the facade of civility, and that was so threatening to everyone that it had to be denied once again.

Five years on from that initial piece in which my thinking was challenged at every point, I have come back to or forward to thinking what I wrote then. That is to say, we cannot bear to take on the reality of childhood sexual abuse because it is so awful, so undermining, so emblematic of the deep cultural crisis that we are in. We prefer not to think of it, not to believe it, not to envision that such practices are part of our cultural life. If we accept that they are, then we have to re-draw the way in which we understand human relationships. We have to extend our analysis to account for the frequency rather than the deviance of these practices.

* * *

Let us look for a moment at the impact of secrecy in both the public and the private domain and how in the individual situation this has a bearing on the psychic structure of a woman who had been abused as a child.

Part of why so much of this only reluctantly comes out in the clinical situation is that it keeps the secret of the original abusing relationship, in which the perpetrator made it clear to the victim that the activities that he (or she) engaged in were never to be revealed. The need to keep a secret, the very fact that the abuse could not be disclosed, has meant that the abused person has had to find a way to cope with this traumatic experience in an abnormal way. Usually, if we are traumatised by a death or an accident or a mugging, we try to work through that experience both cognitively and affectively. That is to say, we try talking about it, we endeavour to understand it and we go through a process in which mourning, rage, grief, horror, terror and so on are experienced in a reasonably supported context. Not so with sexual abuse. The very fact that the person was sworn to secrecy or knew by the emotional ambience of the surrounds of the abuse that secrecy was an important element of it, and the fact that there was indeed no one to turn to who would listen to an account of the abuse and stop it, means that, for many survivors, by the time they get to adulthood they have had to banish it from their conscious or aware self or they will be driven mad by the pain and knowledge of what they have lived through. Their psyche needs to accommodate two concurrent phenomena. First, it needs to find a way to deal with deeply destructive experiences. Second, it needs to find a way to conceal the knowledge of these experiences from others.

What becomes obvious in working with survivors is that much of their life has to be lived in their head because the outside world is a very dangerous place. It is as though they have had to withdraw energy from the real people and relationships in their lives and try to construct scenarios that make plausible, make comprehensible, the fact of the abuse that they have experienced. When the psyche cannot deal with excruciating pain directly, when it cannot speak of it, it has to find ways to account for what has happened that leave the person functioning. One of the ways it does this is that it creates an inner world in which things work out rather differently. There are several processes at work which I will mention because they impact upon the kinds of problems that can occur in the therapeutic relationship.

The first of these processes usually involves the person who has been abused rewriting the events in such a way as to place himself or herself as the central actor in the abuse, that is to say, renders himself or herself as culpable, as though he or she were somehow at fault for what has happened or is happening. Now this may seem bizarre – that the victim turns herself or himself into an instigator – but if we think of the feelings of powerless and helplessness that we all find incredibly difficult and we multiply them several-fold, and we imagine ourselves to be living in a situation that is already too dangerous to disclose and so we are insecure to begin with and have the experience of being disregarded, we can see that a psychically lethal combination of low self-esteem and the psyche's inability to contain feelings of defencelessness creates a push to escape in fantasy from the situation by creating a scenario that has a get-out clause – in other words, by making oneself somehow at fault. If one is at fault, then one could somehow find a way to stop. One is potentially powerful rather than powerless. This reversal of what is, momentarily soothes the pain of powerlessness and creates a sense in the person that he or she is not without resources or possibilities for escape.

Now the difficulty with this scenario – apart from, of course, its inaccuracy and the harm that it does the person – is that in a therapy relationship this survival mechanism, this taking on of the fault, is very hard to dislodge. The reason is that in order to dislodge it one is asking the client to give up the defence that she has constructed, one is suggesting that she can manage the despair, helplessness, rage and so on that has been repressed, and she, of course, does not feel that she can. In the therapy, in wishing to respect the client one can also feel as though one is tempted to engage in a tug-of-war, with the client inviting one in, as she discloses a little, and then her shutting the therapist and herself out as she reconstructs the scenario in which she is an instigator. This is a frustrating process because good therapeutic practice demands that she be able to feel, to take on board her experience of the abuse, at a pace that is manageable.

As a therapist one may wish to be more powerful in return, so that when we say "Look, this happened to you and you were vulnerable, and you couldn't do anything about it, and that is what we have to face together, the fact of what happened, the pain of what happened and so on", we want to be doing magic. We want our words to clear away the psychic distortions that she has created, but they can't, and so we too feel deeply impotent.

Allied to the taking on of culpability is the identification that many survivors unconsciously make with their abusers. In its most extreme form, it is as though there are sub-personalities to the survivor which she may or may not know about. They may emerge during the course of therapy, so that at one moment or in part of a session one will be dealing with an aspect of self who is a compliant or sweet little girl, at another with a dissociated part who is an angry, wilful, destructive little witch, or else a hateful, abusive, and manipulative part. None of these part selves or separate personalities are necessarily truer than others. There may be a central self that complies with social norms, keeps down a job, looks after the kids, and so on, but there may be subsidiary selves, known or unknown to the central self, that undermine and ridicule whatever she is able to achieve (Davies & Frawley, 1994; Herman, 1992).

Now the difficulty for the therapist is that first he or she may not know about these separate selves for a long time, and when they do come out they may break all conventional boundaries in ways that the therapist feels unprepared for. They will press demands on the therapist for extra kinds of caretaking, which invite a breaking of therapeutic boundaries. I am thinking here of the pressure on the therapist to see the person several extra times a week, take telephone calls at ungodly hours, let the person move into the therapist's own home, give her money and so on. These kinds of pressures are not uncommon for therapists working with survivors of sexual abuse. If there is a place to discuss the pressure that the therapist feels under, then he or she will be more able to provide a creative answer; often, however, the therapist gets drawn into a feeling that the urgency of the client's situation is misunderstood and that colleagues are being too rigid, and so the therapist withdraws from talking about the pressure, accedes to breaking boundaries in an unhelpful manner and then becomes drawn into the client's drama in such a way that he or she is forced eventually to disappoint her, prove untrustworthy and reiterate at a psychological level the experience of being let down that the client needs to work through rather than re-enact.

The pressure to re-enact at an emotional level is, of course, part of what occurs in any therapy, and that pressure and the ability to understand it and work through it with the client is central to the process of therapy. With survivors, where the pressure is so forcefully turned up, it is crucial that there are supervisory sessions where this pressure can be discussed rather than the therapy becoming a secret re-enactment or acting out.

I was saying that one of the psychic consequences of the splitting-off of indigestible experience is the identification that the client may unconsciously make with her perpetrator. This identification can have many forms, but the particularly troublesome ones occur when the therapist feels as though she or he is being abused in the therapy relationship. This is a difficult thing to talk about, but it does seem to be a reasonably common occurrence in therapy, and many therapists and workers, if given half a chance, talk about feeling guilty and confused about their experience of feeling abused and used by the clients. It is not in the actual things that are said but in a kind of emotional ambience that they feel is created in which the therapist comes to feel through the process of projective identification a version of what the client felt. The client finds an emotional way to communicate what she felt and feels at a nonverbal level about being abused. Along with the capacity to arouse these feelings in the therapist, there is also a counterpart in that the therapist can feel sadistic in return and can identify with the sadism and cruelty of the perpetrator. We are now learning that such feelings and responses are perfectly expectable in therapy with people who have survived what seems like the unsurvivable.

In our work with survivors, we face many problems. A consequence of the abuse is that the person we are working with may never have experienced relationships that are not marked by abuse; alternative relationships, relationships that are not characterised by abuse, have very few psychological channels to go down. In other words, if the relationships on which a person is meant to rely have forsaken her in treacherous ways, then she learns that relationships are perilous. So if mother has betrayed us by allowing our father, brother, step-father, uncle, grandpa, neighbour to abuse us consistently, or if mother herself has been a perpetrator of abuse, then we understand that relationship means abuse. We do not have an alternative emotional framework. We may read about hearts and flowers relationships, see them on television, but our own imprinted experience is of betrayal. But this betrayal, with the meagre relationship it offered, may have been the only relationship that was given to us, so to desert it, to abandon the structure of this kind of relationship, to disavow this form of relating, is almost impossible because as the model for relationship and the central relationship it is still desperately needed.

This need and this pattern then shapes other relationships, so that when a relationship that is not abusive is offered – such as a therapy relationship – it may appear to the person as abusive; and if it does not turn out to be abusive, the person may find herself so confused that she tries to shape this relationship in line with relationships that she has known. The struggle to reshape what relationship can mean, the need to bear witness to profound horror, the attempt to help the survivor put the culpability where it really belongs, the need to resist the narcissistic pull to be the one person who can save this person's life all make working with survivors both very difficult, very moving and profoundly rewarding. But to do it we need to be listened to as well. We need mini-versions of the space that we give our clients, so that we can process together the horror that we have learnt about without repressing it in turn.

Sexual abuse is a horrifying aspect of daily life for many people. It constitutes a war on our children, it pollutes their lives, and it exercises a chilling effect on the rest of us. I, for one, would rather not believe it. I want to deny its prevalence and reserve its particular horror as the misfortune of the few. I want to applaud and valorise those who survive. Like anyone else, I want the stories to be inaccurate; emotionally, I wish that false memory were a phenomenon that I could believe in. It would relieve me of the burden of accepting the wide-scale nature of child abuse. But I can't. Yes, false memory can occur; yes, there are rotten therapists and so-called healers out there. But to focus on that is to discharge us of the responsibility of understanding the conditions that create sexual abuse and absolve us of the need to work to change the structure of relationships that produces them.

I am at a loss to understand how sexual abuse can occur on such a wide scale, but I do accept that it does. I cannot theorise the whys. I can only comment on the practice and the reactions that I observe in those who have been abused – as well as the reactions of us who haven't – to the fact of abuse. In my incomprehension, I struggle to understand the clinical implications and consequences of abuse. I know that others, some of whom are workers in the field of sexual abuse, are better able to theorise the whys. But just because we find it hard to accept and hard to comprehend, it does not mean that we should take the easy way out and focus our attention on something that we can get a hold of – false memory. That is a problem, to be sure. But we need to devote our efforts to confronting why we, as a culture, can tolerate the sexual abuse and torture of children.

References

Davies, J. & Frawley, M. (1994). *Treating the Adult Survivor of Childhood Sexual Abuse. A Psychoanalytic Perspective.* New York: Basic Books.

Herman, J. L. (1981). *Father-Daughter Incest.* Cambridge, MA: Harvard University Press.

Herman, J. L. (1992). *Trauma and Recovery.* New York: Basic Books.

Masson, J. (1984). *Freud: The Assault on Truth.* London: Faber & Faber; New York: Farrar, Strauss, Giroux.

Hoggart, S. (23 March2004). *The Observer.*

Sinason, V. (Ed.) (1994). *Treating Survivors of Satanist Abuse.* London: Routledge.

Chapter 8

Trauma, skin: memory, speech

Ann Scott

In this chapter, from the original *Memory in Dispute* (Sinason, 1998), Ann Scott looks at the role of language and speech in the false memory debate. Drawing on the psychoanalytic work of Henri Rey, she provides a careful linguistic analysis of the pain involved in this subject. At the end of the original piece Ann Scott adds an update.

One of the first features to strike us when we consider the question of false memory and the controversy that it has generated is the role of speech both in organising the terms of the debate and in preserving the anguish for those involved, in both generations of the families. I use a word as strong as anguish deliberately: the briefest survey of the ephemera of the False Memory Syndrome Foundation shows how much pain is embedded in the letters and statements of those who feel themselves to be falsely accused (see for example, FMS, 1993). Because it is increasingly recognised that sexual abuse is a profound impingement of boundaries, psychic and actual, we tend to react with anger to a "denial of the truth" on the part of a parent accused of abuse (who is most likely, of course, to be the father). But I want to suggest that it is in the nature of this situation as a whole – where memories are so much at odds – that words can, to cite Henri Rey (1986, p. 185), "be expelled as unwanted objects", by both daughters and parents. Furthermore, since sexual abuse and the memories associated with it concern the body, I want to suggest that it is through considering something about the relationship, felt and linguistic, between words and the subjective sense of the skin as the body's boundary that we might be able to account for at least some of the uncontained feel that this debate has come to have and the experience of puzzlement that many have at the irreconcilably different accounts of the family members involved. My text is the reported speech of concerned journalism, and I am examining the issue through the lens of an idea about dialogue evolved within the clinical setting.

Let us assume, first of all, that the memory of a trauma can be recovered – as the British Psychological Society's survey data suggest (Morton et al., 1995) – then what strikes us in the situation is how violent the debate around false memory syndrome has become. Here it may be important to note that whether or not sexual abuse is known to have taken place – indeed, whether or not it may

DOI: 10.4324/9781003193159-9

have taken place, is being denied by the accused parent (who knows consciously he committed the acts) or is being denied by the accused parent (who is genuinely in denial), has been remembered all along by the daughter, or had been unknown and then remembered in adult life – a cultural taboo is being violated at the level of language, if not at the level of the body. For one of the paradoxes about the discourse of incest at the moment is that even though transgressions of the incest taboo are now increasingly accepted as widespread in practice, the taboo as a cultural requirement continues to exercise its demands. So, something unthinkable is seen to have been thought; and, because it is seen as the unthinkable, its expression in words is met with aggression.

Beatrix Campbell demonstrates beautifully, to my mind, how this process shows itself in the culture, in her fine account of three cases where abuse was denied (Campbell, 1995). Although her purpose is to subvert the false memory argument by showing that in these particular cases the abuse had been spoken of by the young women before they had had any therapy – so that what was in play was not recovered or false memory at all – her article illustrates very well the level of hostility, fear, disruption, and disturbance that such words and memories are bound still to elicit. The language is, strikingly, one of warfare as mediated by the journalist's voice. Let me quote just one of her vignettes: a daughter and her mother, in

> a middle-class family whose usual unhappiness has been detonated by a young woman in her 20s whose way of living with herself is self-destruction, starvation and attempted suicide. The daughter has always known why she was trying to die. When she tells her story her body buckles, her voice fades and the blood drains from her taut face. Despite her difficulty, and despite her mother's disbelief, her narrative is crisp and eloquent.
>
> (p. 27)

The wife insisted that her husband and her father could not have abused her daughter:

> She rages, she weeps, she harangues her daughter's hospital, she has become a procedural vigilante, she keeps voluminous files of correspondence with the health and social services. She claims her daughter got her ideas from books, from other patients, from dreams, but not from her own experience. She fires false memory syndrome literature at the young woman. Their conversations are consumed by it.
>
> (p. 28)

Both these women's words are unwanted by those to whom they are addressed. Because the experience is contested – as the title of the original book, *Memory in Dispute* (1998), reminds us – those involved are left with unusually raw, unheard words and the impassioned reactions that they evoke, as are we, the readers. How might we think about such angry sequences? Very speculatively, I want to suggest that Henri Rey's work on psycholinguistic structures (Rey, 1986) may offer a helpful starting point for at least some of the exchanges that are in play. I do not overlook the difference of setting, and it could be argued that the two registers – clinical and journalistic – are too different to be discussed in this way. On the other hand, the media's concern with false memory syndrome (an extension of its concern with sexual abuse generally) has been on a scale that invites deeper consideration and may be helped, I am suggesting, by ideas evolved within the clinical setting.

Rey's general argument is that sounds normally become words through projective identification, and that words can be seen as objects: the argument builds up slowly, and I can only quote selectively from it:

> [T]he sound-word – the sound becoming a word as it acquires domain (meaning) – is at the same time acquiring an inside space, like we have seen for other objects. This *inside of words, or words as containers*, is brought to our attention through a great number of expressions in the language ... Phenomena of displacement and condensation, achieved by projective and introjective identification, structure objects. Words are similarly structured. Experiences are projected into sounds, making them words by projective identification. Thus when words are used, *they evoke the experiences they contain*.
>
> (Rey, 1986, p. 184; emphasis added)

The suggestion, then, is for words to be seen as "structured like any other objects" (p. 183), and as being "used for the interiorization of experiences or structures, and the fixation of these experiences in memory" (p. 185). These ideas can act as a marker, in my view, in making sense of the quality of the disputes around false or recovered memory. For here it is an *un*certainty or elusiveness of experience, terrifying for those involved, which permeates everything: words, memory, violation of bodily and psychic space – all seem to have become rootless, mobile; the words seem to lack an inside space, at least as they are reported by the journalist.

We might also speculate that this "inside space of words" is normally paralleled – or even made possible – by the sense of inside space that is created by the skin as a boundary between inside and outside. Where abuse has taken place, or is *felt* by the subject to have taken place, the sense of disturbance in the continuity of the skin as a boundary may make words less stably present for him or her. In the special case where memory is beginning to emerge in adulthood, the words have no history of being bound to an experience of which the subject is confident. So, what is likely to happen when an adult daughter is faced with the dilemma of attempting to communicate, within her family, what she now, however tentatively, believes is a memory of something actual that happened – which at the same time would represent the violation of a taboo that is part of the cultural and linguistic context in which all are placed? My suggestion is that her words become "unwanted objects", and in that process their volatility is assured.

To amplify: Rey attempts first, as I have mentioned, to map the nature not of this type of highly charged communication in particular, but of the relationship in principle between speaker and listener in any exchange. Taking up René Thom's work, Rey focuses particularly on the concept of "semantic density", which, broadly, grades words according to their volatility when they are spoken (Rey, 1986, p. 181). The account of the semantic density of different parts of speech is somewhat technical but could, I think, be imaginatively invoked in situations of newly remembered abuse to make sense of a phenomenon that is a puzzling feature of some (but not all) recovered memory narratives: the susceptibility to retraction, the evaporation of conviction when daughters take back their accusations. I should stress that here I am concerned only with those cases where the impasse across the generations is maintained; not where daughters have, over time, come to believe their memories were not reliable and a reconciliation has been achieved.

On the face of it an overly chemical term, the notion of "evaporation" may shed light on the paradoxical disparity seen in some of the cases: between a sufferer's continuing symptoms and the change that her speech may undergo. Take the charge "You abused me" or "My father abused me", later retracted – what is at work when such a conviction is given up? (My stress is on the exchanges reported in the many media accounts, not on the clinical exchanges in which the "You" may refer, in the transference, to the analyst.) According to Rey, here focusing on the elements of speech themselves, a verb will in principle be more "volatile" than a substantive, and, in a transitive sentence, the object will be more volatile, less semantically dense than the subject – that is, certain words will disappear, others remain in place. Could the concept of semantic density help us to map the volatility of the communication we often see in media accounts of false or recovered memory dynamics? I am suggesting that if the words are not held by their recipient (and it is not surprising that they are not), they function as "unwanted objects" and are less likely to remain stable for the one who speaks them.

In these dynamics it is painfully clear that resonance between speaker and recipient is lacking; there is no linguistic communication. In the sentence "You abused me", for example, the verb would be the most volatile, then the object, while the subject – here, the father – would crucially remain in place. Again, the other's "flat denial" might lead to an evaporation into thin air of the most volatile elements of the subject's memory, leaving the speaker utterly bereft of confirmation and vulnerable to retraction. The troubling ending that Campbell (1995) leaves us, her readers, with highlights the point. Why has the young woman whose abuse was denied gone on to make another suicide attempt? Could it be born of a fantasy? Who put the memories into her head? "Nobody did but me", she says in her retraction (p. 28). The reader is understandably disturbed by the apparent volte face. But as Campbell writes – tellingly, to my mind – "the syntax if not the substance of her story" had changed (p. 28).

This is not to say, on the other hand, that the resolution of the daughter's pain would depend only on her father ultimately affirming her experience. That would be to ignore the psychic processes at work in him, and also to assume that reliability of memory is itself a straightforward matter. Indeed, it may be a mistake to treat the issues raised by the false memory controversy as though they were of a different order altogether from those raised by sexual abuse that has always been remembered. In individual cases, of course, the situations will be different: since it is increasingly accepted that sexual abuse can be damaging at many levels, one might expect more uncertainty about the effects in cases where memories begin to emerge in adult life but in fact remain very shadowy. Symptoms may be more nebulous. From another angle, however, a clear distinction between "actual" and "imagined" may also be becoming harder to maintain. Parental behaviour that may have been intrusive, though falling short of actual abuse, may appear as memories that have metaphorical rather than literal truth (cf. Mollon, 1995; see also Chapter 10, this volume). Also, as Lesley Stubbings, who sued for compensation after the memory of her abuse returned in adulthood, said in a television interview: "When you're a child you haven't got a vocabulary. You don't think 'I've been violated'" (First Sight, 1995).

At source, sexual abuse – whether real or imagined, always known, or reconstructed in adulthood – involves the skin and feelings about the skin and its sensations early in life, for before there is adult speech there is the bodily experience – actual, imagined or metaphorical. Here is Linda, an adult woman in a sensitive television documentary, recalling early sexual abuse, remembered as an adult; she is shot in close-up and framed so that her eyes are not visible, and we see only her nose, mouth, and chin. The aggressive editing of the image enhances the effect of her words:

> This thing in my mouth ... a shape ... I started getting this choking feeling- and somehow I knew it was a penis ... a razor blade close to my chest.
>
> (First Sight, 1995)

These are not the benign, nurturant skin sensations that Esther Bick described as giving evidence of a containing object – the joining of nipple and mouth (see Bick, 1986; Hinshelwood, 1991) – but the malign, confusing skin contact that disrupts peace and safety. Here we could say that the father's skin has failed to be the skin that the infant-child needs. Again, very speculatively, we might take Bick's picture of the object that fails to contain (and, by extension, the internal containing object that fails to contain) as being felt as a partial skin, as tending to develop holes, and link it, forwards in time, with the daughter's psychic predicament. Here her own skin feels "partial" and her words have come to lack their inside space. I am suggesting that the skin contact of father and daughter has had its primitive traumatic effect.

In some cases, of course, the sense of the early experience will only be recovered in adult life; where this is then denied by the parents, the adult daughter is faced with a psychic gap, a further lack of containment: the original trauma is compounded by the trauma of a denial. The daughter's words, which lack their inside space because of disturbance in the boundary of the body, lack stability.

Her situation is, I am suggesting, reminiscent of that of the infant where the primitive skin contact has "leaked". Bick, to quote Eric Rhode (1994),

> concentrates on aspects of infancy in which there is a falling apart or a leaking of a provisional holding-together.
>
> The infants exist as actions in a nowhere that is everywhere ... Their feelings derive from sensations: they have little sense of internal *figures* to whom they might relate.
>
> (p. 270)

To extend this point, one might suggest that the words go into or come from a kind of limitless space. As one mother said, "I don't know where these false memories are founded", and yet she is certain that "these amazing allegations came out in therapy" (quoted in Campbell, 1995, p. 27). With this we are brought back to the virulence that is in play. I come to a final point: that the sense of danger is felt not just by those who are accused. As Rey (1986, p. 184) says, words can be felt as "dangerous objects inside" as well, so the accuser feels guilty about the accusation too. And just as Rey describes a patient who simulated suicide many times in order to have her stomach washed out, "because she said that words were mouldy, poisonous, dangerous objects inside her stomach, and if she talked they would hit the therapist and do him great harm" (p. 184), so memory may not always be benign – far from it. Campbell (1995, p. 28) describes an incident in which one young woman saw something in a Christmas catalogue that reminded her of her baby brother being abused with a toy. "It was a memory she hated having", she says baldly and movingly.

I have been suggesting that the "trauma of false memory" is a crisis at the level of speech as well as a crisis at the level of the body. Let me end, by way of contrast, with an example from the more crafted language of poetry. Emily Dickinson's lines "The Body – borrows a Revolver – /He bolts the Door", from her poem "One need not be a Chamber – to be Haunted" (Dickinson, 1863, p. 333) also indicate how powerfully productive, and yet violent, words can be in representing sensations at the level of the body. We can recognise, however, that despite the sense of exposure – and danger – in the words chosen, the addressee is in no sense implicated as accused. By contrast, the speech of the adult daughter who recovers memory has gone further and is sometimes (and understandably) accusatory. Yet it is a form of speech which in the nature of things may act as an "unwanted object" to its recipient and, because of that, circulate in an uncontained space. Interestingly, as we know, some of those who have recovered memories have not sought to confront their abusers or, ultimately, take legal action. They have intuitively preferred to allow the memories to stay inside. And if they are able to maintain the sense of an "inside space" that is safe, their healing may perhaps prove more stable.

Acknowledgements

I am very grateful to Valerie Sinason, Lesley Caldwell, Bob Hinshelwood, Meira Likierman, Marilyn Pietroni and Jean Radford for their help and comments on a first draft of this chapter; and to an informal seminar around the paper in September 1996, organised by Prophecy Coles.

2020 update: postscript

In "Trauma, skin: memory, speech", I wrote about a cultural crisis at the level of speech, in which daughters' narratives of abuse were vulnerable to retraction. Twenty years later, we are witnessing another crisis in relation to sexuality, but this time speech is more stable, and indeed culturally validated. In the UK the statutory Independent Inquiry into Child Sexual Abuse, established by the government in 2015, includes a Truth Project for victims and survivors "to share their experiences in a supportive and confidential setting", emphasising that they "make an important contribution to the work of the Inquiry". #MeToo and Time's Up, movements opposing sexual misconduct and harassment in the wake of allegations against the film producer Harvey Weinstein, gathered momentum at the end of 2017 through the collective solidarity of women's speech. There has been no "evaporation of conviction" as there was in the false memory narratives. On the face of it, both are a measure of how much has changed, in the debate about sexual abuse, sexual harassment and sexual assault. At the same time, we need to remember the difference between private and public space; between the family and the workplace; perhaps, too, a difference at the level of the psyche between the impact of incest, on the one hand, and of harassment and assault, on the other. There is a taboo on incest, with proscribed relationships codified in law that is designed, in part, to protect the sexual boundary between the generations. By definition, the existence of a taboo makes speech more difficult. While there may be – and indeed has been – a silencing of women's experience in the workplace, the relationships involved have not been blood relationships; this may make organised opposition, when it emerges, a more stable possibility. Of course, there is permeability: the IICSA website, while focusing on "claims against local authorities, religious organisations, the armed forces and public and private institutions – as well as people in the public eye", acknowledges that the individual may have been abused by a family member. And there is continuity. The Truth Project makes use of the same visually powerful editing in its invitation to give testimony that was used in the TV documentary I referred to: close-cropped images of a nose, a mouth and a chin, this time captioned "I will be heard" (with a clickable button: "Get in Touch"). But differences remain.

https://www.truthproject.org.uk/i-will-be-heard

References

Bick, E. (1986). Further Considerations on the Function of the Skin in Early Object Relations: Findings From Infant Observation Integrated Into Child and Adult Analysis. *British Journal of Psychotherapy*, 2 (4), 292–299.

Campbell, B. (1 February 1995). Mind Games. *Guardian Weekend*, 23–28.

Dickinson, E. (1863). *The Complete Poems of Emily Dickinson*. Thomas H. Johnson (Ed.). London: Faber and Faber, 1970.

First Sight. (16 February 1995). *False Memory Syndrome*. BBC2 television documentary.

FMS. (1993). *FMS Foundation Newsletter*, 2 (8). Philadelphia: False Memory Syndrome Foundation.

Hinshelwood, R. D. (1991). Esther Bick. In *A Dictionary of Kleinian Thought* (2nd ed.). London: Free Association Books, pp. 230–231.

IICSA. (n.d.). https://www.iicsa.org.uk/

Mollon, P. (December 1995). Clinical Psychologists, Recovered Memory and False Memory. *Clinical Psychology Forum*, 86, 17–20.

Morton, J., Andrews, B., Bekerian, D., Brewin, C., Davies, G. & Mollon, P. (1995). *Recovered Memories·: The Report of the Working Party of the British Psychological Society*. Leicester: British Psychological Society.

Rey, H. (1986). The Psychodynamics of Psychoanalytic and Psycholinguistic Structures. In *Universals of Psychoanalysis in the Treatment of Psychotic and Borderline States: Factors of Space-Time and Language*. J. Magagna (Ed.). London: Free Association Books, 1994, pp. 176–189.

Rhode, E. (1994). *Psychotic Metaphysics*. London: Karnac.

Sinason, V. (Ed). (1998). *Memory in Dispute*. London: Karnac.

Chapter 9

Sigmund Freud's concept of repression

Historical and empirical perspectives

Brett Kahr

In this chapter, the author reviews Sigmund Freud's foundational theory of repression, exploring its clinical relevance. He then considers various experimental psychological research, such as the contributions of Matthew Hugh Erdelyi and Linda Meyer Williams, conducted in subsequent decades, which provides strong confirmatory evidence of the psychoanalytical theory of motivated forgetting.

> Alle Verdräng[un]gen vollziehen sich nähmlich Erinnerungen [All repressions are of memories].
>
> Professor Sigmund Freud, Letter to Pfarrer Oskar Pfister, 10 January 1910 (Freud, 1910b, p. 57; Freud, 1910c, p. 31)

A case of forgetting

On 8 January 1908, a little boy from Vienna called Herbert Graf, aged 4 and three quarters, visited the zoological collection at the Austrian imperial palace at Schönbrunn, accompanied by his mother, Olga Hönig Graf. This particular excursion proved somewhat traumatic and, as the day progressed, little Herbert began to develop a marked phobia of horses. He became fearful not only of stepping outdoors but, also, he fretted that a horse might bite him. The boy's father, Max Graf, a distinguished musicologist, took his son for a consultation with Professor Sigmund Freud, who encouraged Herr Graf to treat the young child according to the new insights of psychoanalysis. Freud himself supervised this pioneering venture in child analysis, and, within a matter of months, Herbert's symptoms abated considerably. Eventually, Freud (1909) published the details of the case, changing the name of the patient from little Herbert to the immortal "kleine Hans" ("Little Hans").

Some 14 years later, in the spring of 1922, Herbert Graf, now a robust lad of 19, visited Freud and explained to the professor that although he eventually came to read the monograph about his childhood phobia, "the whole of it came to him as something unknown; he did not recognise himself; he could remember

DOI: 10.4324/9781003193159-10

nothing" (Freud, 1922b, p. 148).[1] Somehow, Herbert Graf seemed to have obliterated an enormous amount of life experience from his conscious mind. Although the father had recorded a great deal of the small boy's actual childhood speech in painstaking detail, Herbert Graf could recall none of it directly, even after he had read Freud's case history – over 100 pages in length – which might, perhaps, have jogged his memory.

This brief vignette from the annals of psychoanalytical history serves as but one instance which illustrates the very powerful vagaries of human memory.

Freud's writings on repression

For many centuries, the study of memory systems remained a matter of relatively small interest. Across the years, those investigators who had actually written about the subject contributed a range of often outlandish notions about the functioning of memory. For example, during Antiquity, the Greek philosopher Diogenes, who flourished in the 4th century BCE, postulated that the act of forgetting results from a disruption in the appropriate distribution of air throughout the different parts of the body. Many centuries later, the French writer René Descartes hypothesised that disturbances of memory might result from a failure of certain animal spirits to move successfully throughout the brain. By the late 19th century, the burgeoning discipline of experimental psychology provided scientists with new methods for studying memory in a more systematic fashion. Subsequently, large numbers of cognitive psychologists researched this subject even more extensively, generating a significant body of empirical research. But much of this work has remained, by and large, the province of relatively sequestered, academic, behavioural scientists, rather than contributions from mental health clinicians who grapple with the vicissitudes of human memory on a daily – indeed, hourly – basis.

In recent years, the subject of human memory has become a focus of considerable public interest as a result of the heated debates surrounding the so-called false memory syndrome (e.g. Loftus & Ketcham, 1994; Ofshe & Watters, 1994; Hacking, 1995; Wassil-Grimm, 1995). Journalists who have written on this controversy have implied that mental health professionals and research scholars have only recently begun to grapple with the problem of true memory as opposed to so-called false memory. But let us pause to remember that Sigmund Freud had already devoted nearly half a century of sustained contemplation to this very concept. In view of Freud's considered writings on the topic of repressed memory, and in view of the growing body of empirical data which has arisen from Freud's theories, there may well be some merit in examining certain highlights from Freud's vast catalogue of observations on these matters.

The notion of "repression" entered the psychological literature at least as early as the first decades of the 19th century. The German philosopher Johann Friedrich Herbart had already used the word "Verdrängung" – repression – in his writings and, especially, in his book on *Psychologie als Wissenschaft* (*Psychology as Science*), published in 1824, several decades before Freud's birth in 1856. Freud himself first referred to repression in an article written jointly with his colleague Dr Josef Breuer, published in two instalments in the *Neurologisches Centralblatt* – a German-language neurological journal – on "Ueber den psychischen Mechanismus hysterischer Phänomene (Vorläufige Mittheilung)" (Breuer & Freud, 1893a, 1893b), and known to English readers as "On the Psychical Mechanism of Hysterical Phenomena: Preliminary Communication" (Breuer & Freud, 1893c). In reflecting on hysterical patients who had suffered from a psychological trauma, Breuer and Freud underscored the need of certain patients to repress the painful reality of agonising events from their minds.

Initially, Freud often referred to repression and to its cousin, defence, in an interchangeable fashion but, over time, he began to identify other specific mechanisms of defence such as conversion, isolation and projection, and so forth; repression became only one of several possible unconscious strategies for eliminating psychic pain from the field of consciousness (cf. Anna Freud, 1936).

In his monograph on the life of Leonardo da Vinci, Freud (1910a) made a very important contribution to the study of childhood memories. He wrote with tremendous prescience that, with the passage of time, early impressions and memories become modified and that every individual will struggle over the differentiation between reality and phantasy. In recognising the often blurry line between true events and subsequent phantastical revisions, Freud had anticipated virtually every one of the essential debating points in contemporary discussions over false memories, fully recognising the sheer complexity of teasing out true memories, and emphasising that the conscious knowledge of childhood events may readily become repressed, only to re-emerge at a later point in the life cycle. In 1914, in his monograph on the history of the psychoanalytical movement, Freud (1914) had actually referred to repression, quite baldly, as the very cornerstone upon which the whole structure of psychoanalysis rests, ever aware of the vast extent of repressed memories.

By 1915, Sigmund Freud had observed innumerable instances of repression in the course of his psychoanalytical work with troubled patients; he soon published a more clearly articulated theory of this subject in his article on "Die Verdrängung" (Freud, 1915a), known in English, simply, as "Repression" (Freud, 1915b). This brief, but dense, text remains Freud's fullest statement on the subject of repression, and as such it merits a more detailed explication.

Freud began his essay by investigating the ways in which the human organism attempts to protect itself from a painful or an unbearable situation. He conceptualised repression primarily as a flight from an intolerable idea which occurs in the mind. Freud noted that if the unpleasant trigger existed in external reality, such as an attacking lion or a menacing tiger perhaps, then it would be natural to flee; but when that trigger operates internally, then the organism must flee in a mental sense. Sadly, in such circumstances, "flight is of no avail, for the ego cannot escape from itself" (Freud, 1915b, p. 146).[2] Therefore, according to Freud, the ego must condemn a piece of psychological reality and utilise the mechanism of repression to eradicate this data from consciousness. Indeed, he summarised his basic postulate in a succinct manner, explaining that "the essence of repression lies simply in turning something away, and keeping it at a distance, from the conscious" (Freud, 1915b, p. 147).[3] He also underscored that repression tends to be synonymous with the region of mental life known as the unconscious, which becomes the repository of banished or unbearable ideas and affects.

Freud (1915a, p. 130) noted that repression unfolds in two distinct chapters. In the first phase, known as "Urverdrängung" – primal repression – the controversial piece of psychic life becomes obliterated from consciousness. In the second phase of repression, known as "eigentliche Verdrängung" (Freud, 1915a, p. 131) – repression proper – all experiences intimately related to the original repressed piece of the mind undergo repression as well, so that this particular defence mechanism actually infiltrates many areas of life. For example, if a young girl suffers from a traumatic rape by her father and then blocks this memory from her conscious mind, we would refer to this process as primal repression. If, then, some years later, this same young girl, now a woman, should come to engage in consensual sexual intercourse with a male partner, and should find it distasteful but did not know why, we would understand this as a manifestation of repression proper. In other words, all reincarnations of the original repressed event would themselves become subject to further repressions. In severe cases, abused children who then come to have sexual relations during adulthood may even repress adult sexual activities entirely in an effort to eviscerate all physicality from consciousness.

Thus, Freud had hypothesised that the effects of a single act of repression may persist unabated throughout the life cycle. He also indicated, however, that an instance of repression need not be total or comprehensive. Often, only a particular aspect of a certain event will be repressed, and contemporary clinicians might refer to this as partial repression. Freud (1915a) stressed that repression operates in quite an individualistic manner in all cases. Additionally, the utilisation of repression will require a heightened cathexis of the libidinal energy; in other words, the emotional cost of repression will be extensive since we devote so much psychological energy to the maintenance of repressions. In crude terms, Freud had suggested that each of us has to work very hard to remember that we must forget something especially unpleasant.

Sadly, Freud had observed that an act of repression often results in the formation of clinical symptoms. He had already become aware of this finding through his collaborative work with Josef Breuer, but Freud came to expand the theory further, based on the accumulation of additional case material. For instance, in 1918, he provided a clinical example from his treatment of the Russian aristocratic patient Sergéi Konstantínovich Pankéev who developed an animal phobia. Freud (1918) commented that the patient did not really fear animals as such, but, rather, through the mechanism of repression and the further mechanism of displacement, Pankéev evacuated his fear of his own father, and then he came to locate the dangerous aspects of his father onto the animals whom he subsequently came to dread. This observation has had a profound impact upon the psychoanalytical treatment of anxiety states and phobic states, because Freud had suggested to us that whenever we express terror about a certain object the psychoanalyst must actually help the patient to search for the origins of such fears in an earlier, more primitive object, often a family member.

Sigmund Freud also realised that repressions could be lifted as a result of psychoanalytical treatment. In his essay on "Trauer und Melancholie" (Freud, 1917a), better known in English as "Mourning and Melancholia" (Freud, 1917b), he observed that the clinical process of psychoanalysis will frequently activate memories, and, that after treatment has progressed satisfactorily, repressed and unconscious memories will eventually return to the fore of consciousness, no longer subject to the disguise of repression.

The concept of repression would feature throughout Freud's writings until the very end of his career. Indeed, in his final book, *Der Mann Moses und die monotheistische Religion: Drei Abhandlungen* (Freud, 1939a), known in English as *Moses and Monotheism: Three Essays* (Freud, 1939b), he noted, in particular, that traumatic experiences will be particularly receptive to the repression of those thoughts and memories from consciousness and that this act of forgetting might well serve as a protective layer against the dangerous pain of remembering.

The role of repression in the extensive writings of Sigmund Freud defies a brief summary. Peter Madison (1956, 1961) and Barbara Pendleton Jones (1993) have written worthy exegeses about the changing vicissitudes of Freud's concept of repression, and the interested scholar would do well to consult these sources for a more detailed consideration of the matter. For our purposes, we must underscore that, although Freud often changed his theories throughout his lifetime, he never abandoned the basic, foundational concept of repression, and he insisted that his clinical data, derived from extensive work with highly distressed patients, propelled him to persevere with his investigation into the way in which all human beings remove painful thoughts and feelings from consciousness.

Experimental research on repression

For more than 50 years, experimental psychologists have sought to investigate the validity of Freud's theories and psychotherapeutic techniques through the independent means of the psychological laboratory. For instance, in 1967, Ralph Norman Haber and Matthew Hugh Erdelyi, two cognitive psychologists, published a landmark article on "Emergence and Recovery of Initially Unavailable Perceptual Material", based upon a study conducted at Yale University in New Haven, Connecticut (Haber & Erdelyi, 1967). These researchers endeavoured to examine whether the psychoanalytical procedure of free association would actually improve recall memory. According to psychoanalytical practitioners, the art of lying on the couch and free-associating does, indeed, facilitate the expression of hitherto repressed memories; and the subsequent unblocking of repressions thereby aids the recovery of the patient.

Haber and Erdelyi enlisted the co-operation of 40 male undergraduate students from Yale University who had the opportunity to view a slide that depicted a scene from the American South, containing a cotton-gin complex, complete with a loading platform, a suction pipe, a wagon, horses, workers, bales of cotton, various buildings, trees and so forth. The subjects observed this picture for the swift duration of 100 milliseconds (i.e. one-tenth of a second), from a distance of 15 feet. Most people would barely be able to tell what they had observed consciously after having glanced at a certain stimulus picture for a mere 100 milliseconds. The researchers showed this stimulus briefly to the subjects, and then invited them to draw on a piece of paper that they had only just recently seen. Thereafter, Haber and Erdelyi asked some of the subjects to begin free-associating, whereas they invited other participants in the study to play a game of darts instead. Subsequently, Haber and Erdelyi asked all of the students to draw the picture a second time.

After completing the testing, Haber and Erdelyi discovered that those subjects who had the chance to free-associate in-between their first and second drawings revealed a great improvement in their memory of the original southern American scene stimulus, whereas those who played darts did not, by and large, improve. The experimenters concluded that the act of free-associating actually increases the ability to remember material outside of conscious awareness.

With great thoroughness, Haber and Erdelyi rated the drawings for accuracy. After the first round of drawings, the free association sub-group scored 36.0 points on average, whereas the dart-throwing sub-group scored 38.5 points on average. However, after the period of free association, the average score in the free association sub-group increased substantially from 36.0 to 51.8, whereas the average score in the dart-throwing sub-group actually declined, from 38.5 to 32.0, thus suggesting a slight memory decay. The leap from 36.0 points to 51.8 points in the free association sub-group represents a highly statistically significant change. As a result of this work, the authors concluded, "The present study has experimentally demonstrated that genuine recoveries of below-conscious material can and in fact do occur as a result of intervening word-association experiences" (Haber & Erdelyi, 1967, p. 627).

Throughout the late 1960s and 1970s, and beyond, Matthew Erdelyi continued this work, which became known as the "hypermnesia" paradigm. If amnesia represents the forgetting of information, then hypermnesia can be defined, by contrast, as the sudden remembering of previously forgotten or repressed information. In fact, Erdelyi conducted an extensive series of studies, mostly at Brooklyn College of the City University of New York, in Brooklyn, New York (e.g. Erdelyi, 1970, 1990, 1996; Erdelyi & Kleinbard, 1978; Erdelyi & Goldberg, 1979). In his ongoing research, Erdelyi deployed infinitely more complex methodologies, investigating recall memory not only in the laboratory situation but, also, examining the growth of recall over longer periods of time in more naturalistic settings. Together, these publications represent a huge body of empirical research that has continued to support the existence of the hypermnesia paradigm.

David S. Holmes (1990) of the University of Kansas questioned the validity of Erdelyi's work and of much of the other experimental data on the existence of repression, in part, because of the laboratory nature of the research. One could of course argue that a university student free-associating to a southern American scene does not necessarily reflect the situation of a putatively abused patient suddenly remembering details of a traumatic rape after free-associating on the psychoanalytical couch. Nevertheless, Erdelyi's data does most certainly substantiate Freud's claim that repressed material can return to consciousness, simply as a result of talking. Fortunately, since the publication of Erdelyi's work, an even stronger piece of evidence has appeared in the literature, which Holmes and others might regard as more valid and more naturalistic.

Linda Meyer Williams (1994a) of the Family Research Laboratory at the University of New Hampshire, in Durham, New Hampshire, undertook a study of a rather different nature in order to examine whether traumatic events can, actually, be forgotten, and whether such forgetting can, in fact, be documented. Ingeniously, Williams obtained medical records of 206 girls aged from 10 months to 12 years, who attended the emergency room of a certain hospital in the United States of America between 1 April 1973, and 30 June 1975, diagnosed as victims of child sexual abuse. Many of these girls had, in fact, suffered from actual vaginal penetration.

In 1990 and 1991, Williams managed to contact 153 of the original 206 girls, now full-grown women. She invited her research sample to participate in an interview study about "the lives and health of women who during childhood received medical care at the city hospital" (Williams, 1994a, p. 1169). The investigator did not mention child sexual abuse, or the fact that these women had suffered child sexual abuse between 1973 and 1975. Eventually, 129 members of the sample agreed to be interviewed by Williams. The women ranged from 18 years of age to 31 years of age, most of whom belonged to the African American population.

Astonishingly, 38% of the sample of 129 women did not report the abuse, which Williams and colleagues knew, on the basis of hospital records, had, in fact, occurred. Williams of course considered the possibility that these women simply did not wish to talk about such experiences to the interviewer, but she regards this as unlikely, especially in view of the fact that these particular women revealed large amounts of other types of extremely intimate information during the course of their interviews with researchers specially trained in speaking sensitively to survivors of child sexual abuse. Thus, although Linda Williams had strong documentary evidence in her possession, which proved that these women had undergone abuse as children, a large proportion had no conscious memory of the events at all, thus suggesting that they had repressed the memory of painful abuse from conscious awareness, in much the same way that the adolescent "Little Hans" had forgotten all about his visits to Sigmund Freud years previously, during his early childhood. As a result of her research, Williams (1994a, p. 1173) concluded, "These findings suggest that having no memory of child sexual abuse is a common occurrence", thus emphasising the realities of abuse as well as the capacity of researchers to provide documentary evidence to this effect (Williams, 1994b; cf. Loftus, Garry & Feldman, 1994; Pope & Hudson, 1995).

Concluding remarks

The concept of repression does not appeal to everyone. Not only do the supporters of the false memory syndrome question the work of Sigmund Freud and those who have followed in his footsteps but, so, too, do many academic psychologists. For instance, Professor Yacov Rofé (1989), a British-trained academic who progressed to professorships in Israel and the United States of America, wrote a book entitled *Repression and Fear: A New Approach to Resolve the Crisis in Psychopathology*, in which he devoted an entire section to the so-called "Inadequacy of the Psychoanalytic Doctrine of Repression", some 48 pages in length, lambasting Freud for his ostensibly inadequate, unproven contributions.

Although Professor Rofé (1989, p. 12) has argued passionately that Freud's theory of repression deserves little attention and that "this psychoanalytic assumption is of questionable scientific status", his book lacks the clinical emphasis that the father of psychoanalysis relied upon as the very foundation of his writings and his teachings. Certainly, as someone who has worked psychotherapeutically for over 40 years, I have drawn upon Freud's work daily within the confines of the consulting room, and I cannot think of a single patient whom I have encountered who did not repress some early memories, many of which would return to consciousness throughout the course of treatment.

Sigmund Freud suggested that we often forget material from our own biographies in the face of overwhelming psychic calamity. We repress certain painful information in order to protect ourselves from remembering its awful impact. And yet, this material can return to us when we start to reflect upon and talk about our experiences. All of the subjects in Matthew Erdelyi's research improved their memories for various stimuli as they began to free-associate; therefore, why should a patient in treatment not also suddenly remember repressed data during the course of a psychotherapy session? Linda Williams's study has demonstrated that while some women will remember abuse after talking about it, others will not, even though we know that such abuse had actually occurred, thus complexifying the picture quite considerably. The study of human memory function remains an ongoing concern but, at the present time, it seems quite reasonable for clinicians to conclude that it might be possible for repressed events to return to consciousness after long periods of time, and that if our patients begin to harbour doubts about the ways in which their parents or other grownups treated them in childhood, then we ought to listen in a cautious but, above all, a serious manner.

Notes

1   The original German text reads: "erzählte er, sei ihm alles fremd vorgekommen, er erkannte sich nicht, konnte sich an nichts erinnern" (Freud, 1922a, p. 321).

2 The original German phrase reads: "die Flucht nichts nützen, denn das Ich kann sich nicht selbst entfliehen" (Freud, 1915a, p. 129).

3 The original German text reads: "ihr Wesen nur in der Abweisung und Fernhaltung vom Bewußten besteht" (Freud, 1915a, p. 130).

References

Breuer, J. & Freud, S. (1893a). Ueber den psychischen Mechanismus hysterischer Phäno-mene: (Vorläufige Mittheilung). [Part One]. *Neurologisches Centralblatt*, 12, 4–10.

Breuer, J. & Freud, S. (1893b). Ueber den psychischen Mechanismus hysterischer Phäno-mene: (Vorläufige Mittheilung). [Part Two]. *Neurologisches Centralblatt*, 12, 43–47.

Breuer, J. & Freud, S. (1893c). On the Psychical Mechanism of Hysterical Phenomena: Preliminary Communication. In James Strachey and Alix Strachey (Trans.). Sigmund Freud (1955). *The Standard Edition of the Complete Psychological Works of Sigmund Freud: Volume II. (1893–1895). Studies on Hysteria.* James Strachey, Anna Freud, Alix Strachey & Alan Tyson (Eds. & Trans.). London: Hogarth Press and the Institute of Psycho-Analysis, pp. 3–17.

Erdelyi, M. H. (1970). Recovery of Unavailable Perceptual Input. *Cognitive Psychology*, 1, 99–113.

Erdelyi, M. H. (1990). Repression, Reconstruction, and Defense: History and Integration of the Psychoanalytic and Experimental Frameworks. In Jerome L. Singer (Ed.). *Repression and Dissociation: Implications for Personality Theory, Psychopathology, and Health.* Chicago: University of Chicago Press, pp. 1–31.

Erdelyi, M. H. (1996). *The Recovery of Unconscious Memories: Hypermnesia and Reminiscence.* Chicago: University of Chicago Press.

Erdelyi, M. H. & Goldberg, B. (1979). Let's Not Sweep Repression Under the Rug: Toward a Cognitive Psychology of Repression. In John F. Kihlstrom & Frederick J. Evans (Eds.). *Functional Disorders of Memory.* Hillsdale: Lawrence Erlbaum Associates, pp. 355–402.

Erdelyi, M. H. & Kleinbard, J. (1978). Has Ebbinghaus Decayed with Time?: The Growth of Recall (Hypermnesia) Over Days. *Journal of Experimental Psychology: Human Learning and Memory*, 4, 275–289.

Freud, A. (1936). *Das Ich und die Abwehrmechanismen.* Vienna: Internationaler Psychoanalystischer Verlag.

Freud, S. (1909). Analyse der Phobie eines 5jährigen Knaben. *Jahrbuch für psycho-analytische und psychopathologische Forschungen*, 1, 1–109.

Freud, S. (1910a). *Eine Kindheitserinnerung des Leonardo da Vinci.* Vienna: Franz Deuticke.

Freud, S. (1910b). Letter to Oskar Pfister. 10 January. In Sigmund Freud and Oskar Pfister (2014). *Briefwechsel 1909–1939.* Isabelle Noth & Christoph Morgenthaler (Eds.). Zürich: TVZ/Theologischer Verlag Zürich, p. 57.

Freud, S. (1910c). Letter to Oskar Pfister. 10 January. In Sigmund Freud & Oskar Pfister (1963). *Psychoanalysis and Faith: The Letters of Sigmund Freud and Oskar Pfister.* Heinrich Meng & Ernst L. Freud (Eds.). Eric Mosbacher (Trans.). London: Hogarth Press and the Institute of Psycho-Analysis, pp. 31–32.

Freud, S. (1914). Zur Geschichte der psychoanalytischen Bewegung. *Jahrbuch der Psychoanalyse*, 6, 207–260.

Freud, S. (1915a). Die Verdrängung. *Internationale Zeitschrift für ärztliche Psycho-analyse*, 3, 129–138.

Freud, S. (1915b). Repression. Cecil M. Baines & James Strachey (Trans). In Sigmund Freud (1957). *The Standard Edition of the Complete Psychological Works of Sigmund Freud: Volume XIV. (1914–1916). On the History of the Psycho-Analytic Movement, Papers on Metapsychology and Other Works.* James Strachey, Anna Freud, Alix Strachey & Alan Tyson (Eds. & Trans.). London: Hogarth Press and the Institute of Psycho-Analysis, pp. 146–158.

Freud, S. (1917a). Trauer und Melancholie. *Internationale Zeitschrift für ärztliche Psychoanalyse*, 4, 288–301.

Freud, S. (1917b). Mourning and Melancholia. Joan Riviere & James Strachey (Trans.). In Sigmund Freud (1957). *The Standard Edition of the Complete Psychological Works of Sigmund Freud: Volume XIV. (1914–1916). On the History of the Psycho-Analytic Movement. Papers on Metapsychology and Other Works.* James Strachey, Anna Freud, Alix Strachey & Alan Tyson (Eds. & Trans.). London: Hogarth Press and the Institute of Psycho-Analysis, pp. 243–258.

Freud, S. (1918). Aus der Geschichte einer infantilen Neurose. In *Sammlung kleiner Schriften zur Neurosenlehre: Vierte Folge*. Vienna: Hugo Heller und Compagnie, pp. 578–717.

Freud, S. (1922a). Nachschrift zur Analyse des kleinen Hans. *Internationale Zeitschrift für Psychoanalyse*, 8, 321.

Freud, S. (1922b). Postscript. Alix Strachey & James Strachey (Trans.). In Sigmund Freud (1955). *The Standard Edition of the Complete Psychological Works of Sigmund Freud: Volume X. (1909). Two Case Histories ("Little Hans" and the "Rat Man")*. James Strachey, Anna Freud, Alix Strachey & Alan Tyson (Eds. & Trans.). London: Hogarth Press and the Institute of Psycho-Analysis, pp. 148–149.

Freud, S. (1939a). *Der Mann Moses und die monotheistische Religion: Drei Abhandlungen*. Amsterdam: Verlag Allert de Lange.

Freud, S. (1939b). *Moses and Monotheism: Three Essays*. James Strachey (Trans.). In Sigmund Freud (1964). *The Standard Edition of the Complete Psychological Works of Sigmund Freud: Volume XXIII. (1937–1939). Moses and Monotheism. An Outline of Psycho-Analysis and Other Works.* James Strachey, Anna Freud, Alix Strachey & Alan Tyson (Eds. and Trans.). London: Hogarth Press and the Institute of Psycho-Analysis, pp. 6–137.

Haber, R. N. & Erdelyi, M. H. (1967). Emergence and Recovery of Initially Unavailable Perceptual Material. *Journal of Verbal Learning and Verbal Behavior*, 6, 618–628.

Hacking, I. (1995). *Rewriting the Soul: Multiple Personality Disorder and the Sciences of Memory*. Princeton: Princeton University Press.

Holmes, D. S. (1990). The Evidence for Repression: An Examination of Sixty Years of Research. In Jerome L. Singer (Ed.), *Repression and Dissociation: Implications for Personality Theory, Psychopathology, and Health*. Chicago: University of Chicago Press, pp. 85–102.

Loftus, E. F., Garry, M. & Feldman, J. (1994). Forgetting Sexual Trauma: What Does It Mean When 38% Forget? *Journal of Consulting and Clinical Psychology*, 62, 1177–1181.

Loftus, E. & Ketcham, K. (1994). *The Myth of Repressed Memory: False Memories and Allegations of Sexual Abuse*. New York: St. Martin's Press.

Madison, P. (1956). Freud's Concept of Repression: A Survey and Attempted Clarification. *International Journal of Psycho-Analysis*, 37, 75–81.

Madison, P. (1961). *Freud's Concept of Repression and Defense: Its Theoretical and Observational Language.* Minneapolis: University of Minnesota Press.

Ofshe, R. & Watters, E. (1994). *Making Monsters: False Memories, Psychotherapy, and Sexual Hysteria.* New York: Charles Scribner's Sons.

Pendleton Jones, B. (1993). Repression: The Evolution of a Psychoanalytic Concept from the 1890's to the 1990's. *Journal of the American Psychoanalytic Association,* 41, 63–93.

Pope, H. G., Jr. & Hudson, J. I. (1995). Can Memories of Childhood Sexual Abuse Be Repressed? *Psychological Medicine,* 25, 121–126.

Rofé, Y. (1989). *Repression and Fear: A New Approach to Resolve the Crisis in Psychopathology.* New York: Hemisphere Publishing Corporation/Taylor and Francis Group.

Wassil-Grimm, C. (1995). *Diagnosis for Disaster: The Devastating Truth About False Memory Syndrome and Its Impact on Accusers and Families.* Woodstock: Overlook Press.

Williams, L. M. (1994a). Recall of Childhood Trauma: A Prospective Study of Women's Memories of Child Sexual Abuse. *Journal of Consulting and Clinical Psychology,* 62, 1167–1176.

Williams, L. M. (1994b). What Does It Mean to Forget Child Sexual Abuse?: A Reply to Loftus, Garry, and Feldman (1994). *Journal of Consulting and Clinical Psychology,* 62, 1182–1186.

Chapter 10

Terror in the consulting room – memory, trauma and dissociation

Phil Mollon

In this chapter, Phil Mollon explores both psychoanalytic and psychological theories of repression and memory as well as taking us into painful clinical illustrations.

When I completed training in analytic psychotherapy several decades ago, I thought that the task of my work was to analyse the structures and conflicts within the patient's mind as they unfolded within the transference. A few years later, when I worked in a general psychiatric service and tried to help people more damaged than those usually attending a psychotherapy service, the cosy security of that tried and tested way of working was shattered; my sense of reality and sanity was repeatedly assaulted by communications of bizarre and horrifying memories, or apparent memories, for which my training had not prepared me. With these more injured and traumatised individuals, it is as if flashback memory, or memory-like material, violently intrudes, smashing the usual framework, assumptions and epistemological basis of analytic practice.

Let me briefly state my present position, having digested these experiences and reflected at length upon the clinical and research memory literature (see also Mollon, 1996a, 1996b, 2002). I believe the following to be the case. False or pseudo-memories of childhood are possible; true memories of childhood trauma are also possible. A person may be able to avoid thinking about these memories for certain periods (a phenomenon that cognitive therapists call "cognitive avoidance"), and this may be combined with mechanisms of pretence and denial to make the memories unavailable. Later, in response to certain cues, or when in a safe environment, the memories may intrude into awareness; sometimes people seek therapy because memories have begun to intrude. Memory is prone to error; we are continually interpreting and remixing our perceptions of past events. Between the extremes of "true" and "false" memory lies a vast area of uncertainty and ambiguity. One task of the analytic therapist is to tolerate this uncertainty and help the patient tolerate this too. Because it is impossible, as listening and responding participants in the analytic process, not to influence the emerging narrative, it is important to be open to a variety of possible understandings of the patient's history and development. Procedures intended to elicit memories of trauma may be

DOI: 10.4324/9781003193159-11

inadvisable because (1) pseudo-memories may be encouraged and (2) the patient may be retraumatised in the process. Understanding the problems of memory in clinical practice requires the cooperation of psychoanalysis and cognitive psychology.

Psychoanalytic views of trauma and memory

Over 100 years ago, Freud was struggling with the relative importance of reality-trauma and fantasy – and in particular the truth status of recovered memory. For example, in a letter to Abraham in 1907, he wrote:

> A proportion of the sexual traumas reported by patients are or may be phantasies ... disentangling them from the so frequent genuine ones is not easy.
>
> (Abraham & Freud, 1965)

As we know, Freud's attention moved from the impact of actual sexual abuse, and memories of this, to the role of the instincts and fantasy and, in particular, to the Oedipus complex. Blass and Simon (1994) describe the stages in Freud's development and discarding of his original seduction-trauma theories and his painful struggle with issues of evidence and truth. Simon (1992), in commenting on the decline of psychoanalytic interest in actual trauma and sexual abuse, in a paper entitled "Incest – see under Oedipus Complex: The History of an Error in Psychoanalysis", writes:

> I believe much of what Freud had begun to observe and theorise about incest, and much of what he might have elaborated, migrated to the area of the primal scene, the psychoanalytic trauma par excellence.... Primal Scene thus served as a distraction from, or defence against, the further awareness of the trauma of actual sexual abuse of children by parents.
>
> (p. 971)

Meanwhile, Ferenczi continued to emphasise both trauma in the genesis of mental disorder and the modifications of analytic technique, which he felt were necessary to reach these deeper levels of warded-off experience. This conflicted with Freud's position. In a letter to Freud in 1929, Ferenczi summarised his views:

> In all cases where I penetrated deeply enough, I found uncovered the traumatic-hysterical basis of the illness.
>   Where the patient and I succeeded in this, the therapeutic effect was far more significant. In many cases I had to recall previously "cured" patients for further treatment.
>
> (Ferenczi, 1933)

He also complained of a trend in psychoanalysis towards "overestimating the role of fantasy, and underestimating that of traumatic reality, in pathogenesis".

On the whole, analysts who have emphasised actual trauma have been criticised, often fiercely, as Ferenczi was by Freud. Greenacre (1971), in commenting on the response to her earlier writings on pre-oedipal trauma, which were not specifically concerned with incest, wrote:

> The amount of resistance to my findings took me by surprise, especially the attitude expressed several times by colleagues that my work attempted to undermine the importance of the Oedipus complex.

Winnicott's views on the facilitating environment and on environmental failure, written in reaction to the emphasis of Melanie Klein on innate phantasy, stirred controversy and considerable hostility, but they were perhaps more accepted because he was emphasising inadvertent trauma rather than gross and deliberate abuse.

Contemporary analysts still vary considerably over what credence is to be given to suggestions of actual sexual abuse and trauma. For example, a group of analysts who heard material from the following psychoanalytic therapy were quite divided over whether the patient might have been sexually abused or not.

> The patient shows the following characteristics. She frequently experiences terrors that the male therapist will sexually assault her. For this reason, she will not lie on the couch. Instead, she sits in a chair, which she requested be moved near the door for ease of escape. She often insists on leaving the door open so that she can run away easily if the therapist were to attack her. She is very afraid of men generally. She avoids wearing any clothes that might be seen as sexually provocative. Sometimes she enters a dissociative state and reports in a childlike manner experiences of sexual abuse and violent assault. On occasion, she resorts to action and screaming rather than words and will appear to be enacting scenes of sexual assault. She describes what she calls flashbacks of sexual assault – evoked, for example, by the sensation of a toothbrush in her mouth – and she becomes very frightened and flips into a state of dissociation and disorientation. She presented a series of dreams in which men are breaking into the house she is in; in one of these a pole is thrown through the window; in some dreams she develops amazing strength to repel these men – and in one dream she thrusts an umbrella violently down someone's throat. She believes that she was sexually abused as a child, but she has no clear and visual memories of this.

Was she sexually abused or is the imagery of sexual attack a sexualised form of the patient's own violent wish to intrude and to control the therapist, now experienced in projection as coming back at her? It is the question of who thrust the umbrella phallus down whose throat first. Other possibilities were also suggested, but the idea that she may have been literally sexually abused tended to be the least favoured option.

This ambivalence amongst analysts about the reality or otherwise of sexual abuse is mirrored by that amongst patients. Van Leeuwen, in a paper entitled "Resistances in the Treatment of a Sexually Molested 6-Year-Old Girl" (Van Leeuwen, 1988), describes how the impulse to tell may occur in sudden bursts, unexpectedly, and may be followed by retraction and denial. Non-verbal re-enactments were more frequent than verbal disclosure.

Mechanisms of memory and amnesia: what do we really know?

In all the tangle of arguments around the issues of recovered and false memory, there is much intelligent reasoning and a number of relevant studies but precious little firm knowledge when it comes to the mechanisms of memory we encounter in clinical work.

Repression has never been experimentally demonstrated in the laboratory. However, there is nothing novel or implausible about the notion of avoidance, repression or dissociation of memories of trauma and their recovery, whether in the context of psychological therapy or in response to some other life circumstances. It is essentially a matter of motivated cognitive avoidance. Clinical and naturalistic research (as opposed to that based in a laboratory) that has looked at survivors of abuse has indeed found evidence suggestive of avoidance of memory for trauma (e.g. Briere & Conte, 1993; Feldman-Summers & Pope, 1994; Herman & Schatzow, 1987; Loftus et al., 1994; Williams, 1994). Pope and Hudson (1995) have criticised these studies, arguing that independent documented evidence corroborating the "memory" is required to support the concept of repression. Such evidence is reported by Schooler (1994) and Williams (1995). Few in the field deny that motivated avoidance of memory is possible. The debate is about the reliability of recovered memory.

In 1994, two books were published by two memory experts: *Unchained Memories* by Lenore Terr, who is a psychiatrist who has made longitudinal studies of the memory of trauma victims, and *The Myth of Repressed Memory* by Elizabeth Loftus and Katherine Ketcham – Loftus is an academic psychologist specialising in memory research. The books are strikingly similar in style; both highly readable – and both describe the same murder case where the crucial and sole piece of evidence was an adult's flashback memory of her father bludgeoning a child to death. Terr, speaking for the prosecution, argued that there was every reason to believe that the memory was true and claimed that traumatic memories are retained in particularly vivid detail. Loftus, a witness for the defence, disagreed, arguing that there was every reason to doubt the reliability of the apparent memory, and she claimed that her research showed that trauma particularly interfered with the accuracy of memory. The jury believed Terr. Two memory experts, two divergent views.

Commenting on experiments by Loftus and others which indicate ways in which memory can be falsified in the laboratory, Terr (1994) writes, rather dismissively:

Despite the interesting points in the Loftus research, psychological experiments on university students do not duplicate in any way the clinician's observation. What comes from the memory lab does not apply well to the perception, storage, and retrieval of such things as childhood murders, rapes or kidnappings. Trauma sets up new rules for memory. You can't simulate murders without terrorising your research subjects. Experiments on college students do not simulate clinical instances of trauma. And they have little to do with childhood itself.

(p. 52)

Loftus disagrees, arguing that experimental psychologists study the basic processes of memory formation, storage and retrieval, which can be generalised to real life. She emphasises the essential permeability of memory, described as "flexible and superimposable, a panoramic blackboard with an endless supply of chalk and erasers" (1994, p. 3). Actually, I find Loftus to be the more cautious of the two writers, sensitive to the dilemmas of the clinician but emphasising uncertainty in evaluating memory.

Whilst Terr certainly believes that false memories are possible, she argues that if recovered memory is associated with signs and symptoms of trauma, then this is evidence that the memory may contain truth:

If a child is exposed to a shocking, frightening, painful or overexciting event, he or she will exhibit psychological signs of having had the experience. The child will re-enact aspects of the terrible episode and may complain of physical sensations similar to those originally felt. The child will fear a repetition of the episode and will often feel generally and unduly pessimistic about the future ... If on the other hand, a child is exposed only to a frightening rumour ... to the symptoms of another victim of trauma, the child may pick up a symptom or two ... but will not suffer a cluster of symptoms and signs.

(1994, p. 161)

Perhaps so – but the fact that an apparent memory is consistent with a cluster of symptoms and signs does not prove that the particular memory is true. The "memory" could be a fantasy, congruent with a deep schema of the mind but not containing literal truth. Such a memory could be structurally true but literally false.

How is the experience of trauma processed and stored in memory? The theorising of some cognitive psychologists, such as Schactel, Bruner, Postman, Neisser, Piaget, suggests that memory is encoded in different cognitive modes during the earliest months – in enactive and iconic modes, as opposed to linguistic (Greenberg & van der Kolk, 1987). This reveals the possibility of a blocking of the processing of trauma into the symbolic language necessary for cognitive retrieval – so that a person could then experience "unspeakable terror" or "nameless dread" (van der Kolk, 1996). We might also then expect the possibility of the partial reliving of affective and somatosensory components of traumatic memories, without the symbolic and linguistic representations necessary to place the trauma in its historic context. Such partial flashbacks could be reactivated by affective, auditory or visual cues; for example, the way a person may be precipitated into a state of rage and terror whilst having intercourse with his or her partner. The caution must be added, however, that as soon as the attempt is made to create a verbal narrative out of these somatosensory fragments, distortion and confabulation may begin.

A study by Terr (1991) has a bearing on these issues. She found that amongst 20 children with documented histories of early trauma, none could give a verbal description of events before the age of 2 and a half years, but 18 of these showed evidence of a traumatic memory in their behaviour and play; for example, a child who in the first two years of life had been sexually molested by a babysitter could not at age 5 remember or name the babysitter and also denied any knowledge of being abused, but in his play he enacted scenes that exactly replicated a pornographic movie made by the babysitter. In another example, a 5-year-old child who had been sexually and pornographically abused in a day centre between age 15 and 18 months was amnesic of these events but reported a "funny feeling" in her "tummy" whenever a finger was pointed at her; photographs confiscated from the centre showed an erect penis pointing at her stomach.

Terr has studied traumatised children over many years. She finds that recall for "single-blow" traumas in an otherwise trauma-free environment, which she calls Type I traumas, are usually recalled with startling precision and detail. By contrast, Type II traumas, which involve repeated brutalisation, are processed very differently. She writes (1991):

> The defenses and coping operations used in the Type II disorders of childhood – massive denial, repression, dissociation, self-anaesthesia, self-hypnosis, identification with aggressor, and aggression turned against the self – often lead to profound character changes. Children who experience Type II traumas often forget. They may forget whole segments of childhood ... Repeatedly brutalized, benumbed children employ massive denial.
>
> (p. 16)

What Terr seems to mean here is that repeatedly abused children develop generally disturbed minds, within which memory is disrupted.

My own impression is that the fundamental mental defence against overwhelming trauma is dissociation: this is the child flipping into a state of auto-hypnosis, thinking, "I am not here – this is not happening to me", etc. A patient who came to see me specifically claiming a history of ritual abuse could hardly get any words out in our first meeting. Eventually she gasped, falteringly, "It's difficult to speak because I'm not here". When she did in later sessions talk of early experiences of extreme horror, she would refer to her child self as "she". On one occasion, after giving me a very fragmented and incoherent account of an experience of a mock operation in which she had been told that "eyes and ears" with special powers had been placed inside her so that the abusers would always know what she was thinking, saying or doing, she repeatedly muttered the words "eyes no body". It took some minutes for me to grasp that she was telling me that she had gone into a state of dissociation in which she experienced herself as just two eyes without a body. She was gradually able to explain that she had learnt from an early age to get out of her body when she was subjected to extreme pain; in her imagination, she would, for example, escape into a crack in the ceiling, or into a lightbulb – apparently using some kind of spontaneous auto-hypnosis. Often she would tell me of some early experience of abuse and trauma and subsequently have no apparent memory of having told me, although she would acknowledge a memory of the events described.

This material gives just a hint of the ways in which the consciousness and memory of an abused victim may be scrambled with the deliberate intention of creating maximal difficulty in remembering, in telling, and in being believed. If we add to this the possibilities of abuse before language is acquired, confusions induced by the use of drugs administered by abusers (as is sometimes alleged), and the natural intermingling of reality, dreams, and fantasy in the child part of the mind, as well as the unconscious use of images as metaphors, then we can see what a devil of a job we have in sorting out what really went on!

A patient with a dissociative disorder pointed out to me that it is relatively easy to persuade a survivor of childhood trauma that her or his memories are false, because these may be encoded in a dissociated state – so that the main personality does not recognise them as her or his own. If you try to imagine the experience of a fragmented dissociative personality, it is like having other people living inside your body who claim to have certain memories, but you have no way of knowing whether these are true. Moreover, the narrative of abuse may be presented by the patient in a frightened, confused and childlike state of mind dissociated from the adult state of mind – so that no rational and adult discussion with the "narrator" is possible.

A clinical and theoretical tangle indeed! There are many voices in the memory debate, but none who can reliably lead the clinician out of the maze. The more one hears, the more one is confused, as each claim is challenged by a counterclaim. A major report by the American Psychological Association (1996) offers no consensus but degenerates into a bad-tempered argument between opposing "camps".

Trauma, abuse and the sense of reality

A phenomenon that I have observed with a number of patients is that where a person appears to have been repeatedly traumatised in childhood, he or she is often left with an unreliable sense of reality. If asked, the person may acknowl-edge that he or she sometimes has difficulty distinguishing whether something really happened or whether it was a dream. Over time, their account of "memories" of childhood events may vary – perhaps with a recurring theme but with details and persons involved changing; details of one scene of abuse seem to be transposed and remixed to form new scenes, making identification of the true original scene extremely difficult. It is as if repeated childhood trauma may lead not just to repression or other forms of motivated amnesia, as is sometimes suggested, but also to an even more unreliable memory and sense of reality.

Why might this be? One possibility is that if auto-hypnotic dissociation is a primary defensive response to repeated trauma, a person might then become prone to enter hypnoid states of mind in which judgement of reality is impaired. In such a state a person could be auto-hypnotically generating false memory narratives that mix elements of truth and confabulation, just as may happen in "memory" recall in induced hypnosis.

A further possibility is suggested by a bit of Lacanian theory. With regard to the relationship of the mind to the outer world Lacan (1977) postulates three orders or dimensions: the Real, the Imaginary and the Symbolic. The Real is essentially unknowable; for example, a biological need can only be known through an image or a word, but not directly. The Imaginary is the realm of images, fantasies and wish-fulfilments; the world of the dream, which follows the primary process forms of thought. The Symbolic order is arrived at through entry into the shared social world of language and culture; no one can avoid this transition from the Imaginary to the Symbolic without being psychotic. Lacan saw this achievement being structured through the oedipal crisis, through acceptance of the incest taboo and the "Law of the Father", which forbids both mother and child to repossess each other and which therefore represents a fundamental separation between fantasy and reality. The child's identity and sense of boundaries and reality requires that he or she be excluded from the "primal scene" of the parental intercourse.

In the light of these Lacanian insights, what happens if there is incest with the father or if the child is included in the primal scene? It would follow that then there can be no proper entry into the Symbolic, since the "law-giver" is the "law-breaker". There will be no clear sense of where the "law" is situated. Whilst perhaps escaping full psychosis, the person's sense of reality will be defective. He or she will be immersed in the Imaginary, as if trapped in a dream. The boundary between "inside" and "outside" will be unclear. Internal dream and external reality will confusingly intermingle.

Similar problems may arise if there is cult ritual abuse. If we accept the hypothesis that there are indeed perverse cults, then some children may be secretly exposed to bizarre activities that could normally only occur in a dream or nightmare and are totally outside the shared language and culture of society. Such experiences could not be spoken about and therefore could not be given words and would be foreclosed from consciousness. If primitive fantasy and reality meet up in this way, then the outer world becomes identified with an archetype in which the Terrible Mother and the Terrible Father are perceived as real. Again, the barrier between fantasy and reality is blown away.

Clinical illustration

Some years ago, when I knew nothing about ritual abuse, a patient told me of a strange and horrifying event. No "memory recovery" techniques were used. As far as I am aware the patient had not spoken with any other survivors of this kind of abuse, nor read about it. The account that emerged was a surprise and a profound shock, which left me bewildered and confused.

Helen was a 40-year-old schoolteacher of French origin; she was in once-weekly psychoanalytic therapy because of severe and chronic disturbance of affect and interpersonal relationships. From the beginning, she had presented extensive material relating to sexual abuse by her father. There was no "recovered memory" here – she appeared never to have been amnesic for the abuse and even described it continuing into her adult life. There were also minor hints of more peculiar elements; for example, her father's apparent claim to have paranormal powers, her belief that he used to drug her, and memories of a period in her childhood when disgusting objects, including animal limbs, were put through the letterbox (possibly at a time when her parents, now both dead, were attempting to leave the cult they had been involved with). For a long time, these allusions to more bizarre experiences remained obscure.

There were often indications in the transference of early experiences of sadism. She often perceived me as wanting to control her and repeatedly humiliate her. If I seemed to understand her, she felt that this was only in order to gain more opportunity to hurt her and to control her mind. Sometimes she feared that I would somehow be in league with her father. Her experience of the world seemed to be pervaded by cruelty, terror, and her own intense rage.

One session she reported a frightening experience. During the week, she had been opening a jar of spaghetti sauce in her kitchen and had accidentally dropped it; some of the sauce had splashed up the walls. On seeing this, Helen had run out of the kitchen in a state of great terror, feeling that it reminded her of something but not knowing what. Subsequently she had recalled a vivid childhood "memory" of a terrifying scene in the woods – the details of which need not concern us here, except to say that it was of quite a different order to anything that she had described before.

Unravelling of image, affect and narrative

What was I to make of this apparent memory? Had she recovered a memory or constructed a delusion? Whatever the origin of its content, whether in experience or fantasy, this sudden emergence of detailed imagery and narrative seems typical of "flashbacks" of ritual abuse, which are often preceded by much material regarding sexual abuse; the ritual abuse material emerges later, as if unravelling from a different layer of mental storage. The imagery is often highly detailed and shocking, and its occurrence is in itself traumatic and evokes denial; for example, in the session following this, Helen was preoccupied with a wish not to believe her own account. She experienced urges to punish herself, to slash her wrists, and asked me in a childlike voice whether I now wanted her to kill herself. The power of the processes of scrambling or blocking of memory (if that is what it was) in these cases is illustrated by Helen's account of how she and her sister used to have discussions about whether they should go to the police, but they could never remember what it was they were meant to be going to the police about; they knew something had happened but could never remember what. She told me that she felt she had always remembered what had happened but had not before been able to connect the memories with words. Helen described how certain associative cues had in the past triggered terror; for example, her first church communion, and drinking a bowl of lukewarm soup – but she had not been able to make the connection consciously.

There were other features of dissociation in her presentation; for example, she described a split between the one who came to the session and the one who remembered all the horrors when she was alone. Similarly, I noticed that on occasion she would talk in a way that gave no hint whatsoever of ritual abuse and perversion, and at other times her discourse would be filled with allusions to this.

The dynamics of communicating this material

Did I go in search of this material? Did I expect to find it? No. My response to hearing this and similar material has contained elements of shock, disbelief, dread and terror – and confusion – a sense of difficulty in assessing reality. These, I suspect, are typical countertransference reactions to a communicated experience that is like an assault on one's sense of reality.

I experienced the countertransference as one of a split ego state, part of my mind believing the accounts and another part thinking they are preposterous. In this kind of material, there often seems to be an intermingling of elements that are shocking and believable, with those that are unbelievable. Some survivors of abuse networks claim that this is a deliberate ploy to undermine the credibility of witnesses. Inherent in perversion appears to be a delight in confusion and subterfuge, playing tricks with reality and the sense of reality, the interweaving of truth and lies. A quality of "now you see it, now you don't" seems to pervade both the clinical experiences and the criminal investigations.

I am certain that Helen could not have told me about these things until she felt that I could be receptive to them. Moreover, until she told me, she could not tell herself. Her perception of the look of horror on my face when she told me of the events greatly troubled her, and she frequently referred to this in the years following. She complained that I looked so shaken that I was of no help to her in coping with her own reactions. She felt that she must protect me from further trauma, fearing that I would not tolerate more revelations, whilst at the same time needing to know that I could be emotionally affected by her experiences. It was important to show her, through interpretation, that I could bear to hear what she needed to tell me and could think about it with her.

Helen made much progress, but in the later stages of the therapy she was aware of a continuing struggle against forgetting, recognising her own wish to forget. She remained preoccupied with her fear that I might forget – her point being that someone had to remember. She pointed out with great dismay that I did seem to forget some details of the terrible experiences that she described – and when I checked my notes, I realised that she was correct.

Was it true? Did Helen really witness such serious crimes? Are there perverse cults? How could the account ever be corroborated? What is the best way of responding to such an account? How would the therapy have developed if I had disbelieved that there could be literal truth in what she remembered – could she have still got better? I do not know the answer to any of these questions, but I did not disbelieve her – whilst accepting that I could never know objectively the historical truth and that I might be mistaken. On what basis did I believe her account could contain some literal truth, bearing in mind that I have no evidence outside of the consulting room? On what basis do we believe or disbelieve anyone? Could the whole narrative be a gigantic confabulation? If so, what on earth was its source – and what would be the motive behind the production of a narrative that filled the patient with shame and guilt and the therapist with despair?

Epistemological terror

I suggest three forms of terror in the consulting room.

We may experience terror as we empathise with the patient in the reliving of early trauma and terror.

We can also experience terror if a part of the patient is identified with the abusers and attempts to terrorise us, a form of projective identification.

I am also familiar with what I call "epistemological terror". This is the anxiety and anguish that can be felt over the inability to know whether something terrible really happened or is a fantasy – and, contrary to some traditional psychoanalytic views, it does matter. It does matter to a patient's view of self, family, and wider relationships whether her father actually raped her or whether she fantasised that he did.

I have a patient whom I have been seeing for some years. Sometimes she produces material that seems to relate to ritual abuse, and indeed it seems plausible that she was subjected to such experiences – yet neither of us has ever arrived at any conclusion about this. If we grasp the possibility that something terrible was witnessed, or was done to the patient, or participated in by the patient, and if this possibility begins to seem real to both participants, then we face the terror that both patient and therapist might be mistaken, caught up in a *folie a deux*; or if we lean towards the possibilities, on the other hand, that the images of terrible events are like dream images, bearing a metaphorical but not literal truth, and perhaps contain projections of the patient's own destructiveness, then our terror is that we may both be caught in a collusion to avoid the unbearable literal truth. The therapist walks a tightrope. Yet this metaphor is not entirely apt, implying as it does that he or she must stick to the straight and narrow and avoid falling into error. The therapist cannot just stay in some kind of central position of "neutrality" – to do so is not neutrality but a cop-out – but must help the patient explore the possibilities that are thrown up. Parts of the patient which are in terror may need encouragement to speak, may need indications that they will be heard and believed. An expression of seemingly neutral acceptance which covers private scepticism may be perceived by the patient as indicating not a safe emotional environment. The therapist is in an unenviable position here: if he or she does not believe the apparent recollection of trauma, the child parts of the patient will withdraw; if he or she believes the accounts, there could be dangers of colluding with a false memory. I believe that there are ways through this dilemma, but it is a difficult journey. It depends crucially upon not foreclosing the patient's own uncertainty; the patient who is uncertain may endeavour to undo this tension by eliciting certainty from the therapist.

The patient described above who produced images of ritual abuse without our having arrived at any conclusion about its meaning watched a television programme about a trial in the United States of a group of people who were accused of ritual abuse of children in their care. The programme clearly implied that the convictions were flawed because the evidence from the children was contaminated by suggestions from the therapists. The jury had apparently found this an exceptionally agonising trial; some had become ill. The patient felt that the accused were guilty but also felt that the evidence was indeed contaminated. We talked about this as a metaphor for our struggle and ordeal in her therapy; within her mind, there was a prosecuting counsel that wanted to expose abuse, there was a part of her that felt guilty of a terrible crime, there was a defence that wanted to deny the accusation of abuse, a kind of internal false memory society, there were the child witnesses who needed help and encouragement, but whose evidence could then be said to be contaminated by suggestion – and then there was the jury, she and I, struggling to make sense of the evidence and the conflicting claims. Our only advantage is that we are not under pressure to arrive at a premature verdict. Truly, the tolerance of uncertainty is a most crucial and difficult discipline.

It might be argued that a courtroom is not an appropriate metaphor for the process of psychotherapy. But insofar as a court and a psychoanalysis are both attempting to arrive at the truth, then the analogy is apt, especially when criminal offences are being considered. Children and child parts of the adult patient do need to be helped to tell their story and to be listened to in order to recover – but in providing this help we run the risk of contaminating the evidence. In this and other ways, too, our work is inherently and unavoidably hazardous. Damned if we listen and damned if we do not, we can only endeavour to keep our minds (and those of our patients) open and try to hear and continue to think. Psychoanalytic work is a journey of exploration, through memory and fantasy in the fabric of the life cycle, as it interweaves inner and outer worlds. Searching for truth is at the heart of the analytic endeavour – the danger arises when we think we can find and possess the truth.

Perhaps therapy can become the place where our pain is truly witnessed
and our memories are appreciated, even celebrated, as ongoing, ever-
changing interactions between imagination and history.

(Loftus & Ketcham, 1994, p. 269)

(Suggested guidelines for psychotherapists in relation to memory are
offered in Mollon, 1996a)

On re-reading this chapter that I wrote many years ago (Mollon, 1998), I realise there has been little change in my basic knowledge and perceptions regarding
memory. It remains an area of considerable uncertainty and ambiguity.

There is perhaps a tendency for people to be overly confident of their beliefs and
assumptions regarding memory. For example, I read one legal document where the
"expert" asserted that a complainant's early memories were implausible because
they included too much detail. In my view, a memory expert, such as a psychologist, or a mental health specialist, such as a psychiatrist or psychotherapist, have
really very little to say as to whether a particular reported memory is a truthful
representation of an actual event. Mostly, we simply do not know.

The fact of a person believing that something happened during their
childhood does not indicate that it did happen – only that he or she believes it
happened. Similarly, the belief that something did not happen is not an indication that it did not happen. Memory is sufficiently unreliable, and subject to
such a range of potentially distorting factors, that it should be viewed essentially as a subjective feature of our inner life rather than a record of external
reality. Much of the time this subjective experience may contain elements of
objective truth, but often these elements are limited, and sometimes completely absent. A patient once told me that her memory was so unreliable that
she often experienced "other people's memories" – by which she meant that
she might believe a certain event had happened to her, only to be told by a
friend that the "memory" was based on an account the friend had narrated.

On the other hand, there are, in those who present with very disturbed,
incoherent and fragmented minds, parts of the personality whose overwhelming desire is to speak the truth of their experience, whilst other parts of
the personality may disparagingly assert that the alleged events are fantasy.
The psychotherapist is rarely in a position to know the objective truth – by
which I mean the truth that could potentially be corroborated by another
person or recording device if either had been present. In the majority of cases
encountered in the clinic, no such corroboration is available.

There is no obvious reason why human beings would have evolved a highly
accurate narrative memory of events. It would provide no advantage in either
survival or propagation of genes. By contrast we do need good procedural
memory – knowing what to do in order to survive, including how to avoid
situations that have previously proved harmful.

In his book *The Remembered Present* (Edelman, 1989), the neuroscientist
Gerald Edelman, proposes a theory of neural Darwinism and a model of

memory as recategorisation. He theorises that neurons develop networks of sensorimotor coordination through a process of competition and natural selection, as the neural map networks are repeatedly evoked and enhanced through "re-entrant signalling", according to emotional value and basic biological needs. Current situations evoke previously established neural maps – the present is thus categorised in terms of the past – but the present experience also alters the neural maps. Thus, Edelman describes this form of memory as recategorisation. This is quite unlike any view of memory as static information in storage. Memory is a response, of the whole organism, evoked by the activation of previously facilitated global mappings. A past mental and bodily state is brought to bear on a present situation, thereby linking experiences that have felt the same – a model that is very close to the original psychoanalytic concept of transference, whereby the present is perceived in ways that are strongly shaped by the past. From this perspective, there is no necessity for an assumption that memory is an accurate record of past events. Indeed, the very property of being inaccurate in a literal sense may facilitate the ability to generalise and adapt to new situations. Memory as recategorisation may involve a misperception of both the present and past – and yet there is real experience in both past and present.

For me personally, reading my old chapter re-evokes old feelings of anxiety, dread and confusion – remembering again the tales of horror told by some patients in psychiatric services. The details are mostly no longer clear in my recollection – but the sensorimotor feelings and sensations are present. If I tried to present a narrative of a psychotherapy session from 20 years ago it would carry only a vague thematic resemblance to any more objective record. However, the sensorimotor reactions are strong enough for me to know that I choose not to work anymore with those who appear to have suffered severe and repeated interpersonal trauma in childhood.

The empathy required of the psychotherapist can be too much to bear for sustained periods. It is a human limitation in our capacity to assist one another. The epistemological terror and confusion, if we do not surrender to either of the simplifying polarities ("it did happen" or "it did not happen") can be substantial for the psychotherapist, and such burdens will take their toll.

A detailed exploration of the science and clinical phenomena of memory in a psychotherapeutic context is provided in my book on this topic (Mollon, 2002). The vagaries of human memory are both complex and treacherous. My preference is to rest upon the relatively safe ground of acknowledging our ignorance, uncertainty, and continual potential for error.

References

American Psychological Association. (1996). Final Report of the Working Group on Investigation of Memories of Childhood Abuse. Washington, DC: APA.
Abraham, H. C. & Freud, E. L. (1965). *A Psychoanalytic Dialogue: The Letters of Sigmund Freud and Karl Abraham*. New York: Basic Books.

Blass, R. B. & Simon, B. (1994). The Value of the Historical Perspective to Contemporary Psychoanalysis: Freud's "Seduction Hypothesis". *International Journal of Psycho-Analysis*, 75, 677–694.

Briere, J. & Conte, J. (1993). Self-reported Amnesia for Abuse in Adults Molested As Children. *Journal of Traumatic Stress*, 6, 21–31.

Edelman, G. (1989). *The Remembered Present: A Biological Theory of Consciousness*. New York: Basic Books.

Feldman-Summers, S. & Pope , K. S. (1994). The Experience of "Forgetting" Childhood Abuse: A National Survey of Psychologists. *Journal of Consulting and Clinical Psychology*, 62, 636–639.

Ferenczi, S. (1933). *The Clinical Diary of Sandor Ferenczi*. J. Dupont (Ed.). Cambridge, MA: Harvard University Press, 1988.

Greenacre, P. (1971). *Emotional Growth, Vol. 1*. New York: International Universities Press.

Greenberg, M. S. & van der Kolk, B. (1987). Retrieval and integration of traumatic memories with the "painting cure". In: B. van der Kolk (Ed.), *Psychological Trauma*. Washington, DC: American Psychiatric Press.

Herman, J. L. & Schatzow, E. (1987). Recovery and Verification of Memories of Childhood Sexual Trauma. *Psychoanalytic Psychology*, 4, 1–14.

Lacan, J. (1977). *Ecrits*. London: Tavistock.

Loftus, E. & Ketcham, K. (1994). *The Myth of Repressed Memory: False Memories and Allegations of Sexual Abuse*. New York: St. Martin's Press.

Loftus, E., Polansky, S. & Fullilove, M. (1994). Memories of Childhood Sexual Abuse: Remembering and Repressing. *Psychology of Women Quarterly*, 18, 67–84.

Mollon, P. (1996a). The Memory Debate: A Consideration of Some Clinical Complexities and Some Suggested Guidelines for Psychoanalytic Therapists. *British Journal of Psychotherapy*, 13 (2), 193–203.

Mollon, P. (1996b). *Multiple Selves, Multiple Voices. Working with Trauma, Violation, and Dissociation*. Chichester: Wiley.

Mollon, P. (1998). Terror in the Consulting Room. In V. Sinason (Ed.). *Memory in Dispute*. London: Karnac, pp. 126–141.

Mollon, P. (2002). *Remembering Trauma: A Psychotherapist's Guide to Memory and Illusion* (2nd ed.). London: Whurr/Wiley.

Pope, H. G., Jr. & Hudson, J. I. (1995). Can Memories of Childhood Sexual Abuse Be Repressed? *Psychological Medicine*, 25, 121–126.

Schooler, J. W. (1994). Seeking the Core: The Issues and Evidence Surrounding Recovered Accounts of Sexual Trauma. *Consciousness and Cognition*, 3, 452–469.

Simon, B. (1992). "Incest – see under Oedipus Complex": the history of an error in psychoanalysis. *Journal of the American Psychoanalytic Association*, 40 (4), 955–988.

Terr, L. (1991). Childhood traumas: An Outline and Overview. *American Journal of Psychiatry*, 148, 10–20.

Terr, L. (1994). *Unchained Memories. True Stories of Traumatic Memories Lost and Found*. New York: Basic Books.

Van der Kolk, B. (1996). Trauma and Memory. In B. van der Kolk, A. C. McFarlane & L. Weisaeth (Eds.), *Traumatic Stress*. New York: Guilford Press.

Van Leeuwen, K. (1988). Resistances in the Treatment of a Sexually Molested 6-Year-Old Girl. *International Review of Psycho-Analysis*, 15 (2), 149–156.

Williams, L. M. (1994). Recall of Childhood Trauma: A Prospective Study of Women's Memories of Child Sexual Abuse. *Journal of Consulting and Clinical Psychology*, 62, 1167–1176.

Williams, L. M. (1995). Recovered Memories of Abuse in Women with Documented Child Sexual Victimization Histories. *Journal of Traumatic Stress*, 8, 649–673.

Chapter 11

How can we remember but be unable to recall? The complex functions of multi-modular memory

Mary Sue Moore

Empirical evidence of multi-modular human memory systems is reviewed in light of a new understanding of mental processes. The implications of the concept of multiple, differentiated memory systems are explored within a new paradigm. This helps to differentiate between the understanding of what it means "to know" something, as distinct from what it means "to remember".

Introduction

Three related issues are addressed in this chapter: first, substantial empirical evidence of multi-modular human memory systems – evidence that has important implications for understanding the impact of trauma on memory – is reviewed. These research findings must be reconciled with previous conceptualisations that view "memory" as an independent cognitive function capable of being measured in absolute terms.

Second, limitations to traditional experimental approaches to the study of memory are considered in light of a new understanding of mental process. Traditional experimental studies of memory that attempt to determine "exactly how reliable human memory is or can be" necessarily exclude from analysis crucial interactive aspects of brain process, resulting in findings that we now realise have been incomplete at best and erroneous at worst.

The third focus here is the concept of multiple, differentiated memory systems, which has wide-reaching implications for our understanding of what it means "to know" something, as distinct from what it means "to remember". The paradigm-shifting impact of neurobiological research studies substantiating human innate multi-modular memory has major implications for the positions taken by memory theorists in the on-going debate regarding the accuracy of human memory for traumatic experience. The specific impact of this will be considered as a possible influence on clinical and research professionals who have taken increasingly polarised, vehemently defended positions as they attempt to forge a modern definition of human memory.

DOI: 10.4324/9781003193159-12

New technology elucidates new dynamics in brain function

Beginning in the 1990s, neurocognitive research produced empirical findings regarding the nonlinear organisation and interactive complexity of all human brain functions. Previous methods used to measure brain function – as a state of mind rather than a dynamic process – have limited our conceptualisation of the variability and overall capacity of the human mind. Theoretical formulations of these functions generally involved cause-and-effect statements or attempted measurements of an "absolute" capacity. The most widely accepted methods of data analysis were linear. This chapter is an invitation to the reader to consider the profound implications for mental health treatment and human development of nonlinear, interactive formulations of human brain function that recognise physiological process and context as dynamically linked aspects of an irreducible whole. This understanding of brain function as a dynamic, interactive process, along with the concepts of neural plasticity and multi-modular organisation, forms the basis of a revolutionary new theory of human memory.

The conceptual frame described above relies on a complex systems point of view, not just as an option, but as a necessity, if we are to develop an accurate understanding of any brain function. It has become clear that the adoption of a linear, isolated frame of reference when analysing human brain function – in this case, memory – entails distorting that which we are studying to the point of gathering "false or erroneous" data (Grigsby & Schneiders, 1991; Grigsby, Schneiders & Kaye, 1991).

In the following excerpts, the authors describe the irreducible interactive whole constituted by the organism and its environment; these excerpts lucidly argue for the abandonment of the well-practised experimental approach in which a particular function is selected, and experiments are carefully (and artificially) designed to study this process "uncontaminated" by other human processes. As Gollin noted in 1966, "behavior is 'a function of organism and environment, and the proper way to study it is therefore to observe behavior in many organism–environment contexts'" (Grigsby & Stevens, 2000). Given the organism's extreme sensitivity to contextual conditions, even trivial modifications of either the external or the internal environment will often have striking effects on behavioural outcomes.

According to Grigsby and Schneiders,

> Although not a new idea, this emphasis on the importance of contextual variability runs counter to the tendency in behavioural science, where the standard practice in effect has been to regard individuals (or brains) as the sole source of behaviour. *Failure to consider the context may yield misleading or plainly inaccurate conclusions.* [my emphasis] … That living things are embedded in their context is, in practice, an aspect of reality often overlooked by both practitioners and researchers. Although one obviously cannot hope totally to understand the transactions of the organism in its environment, the arbitrary separation of organisms from their surroundings,

which may simplify research design, is nonetheless erroneous ... Surviving successfully over time requires the adequate, automatic (and hence non-conscious) function of a number of systems (modules) that mediate many factors: motivation, accurate perception of the environment, obtaining what is needed for survival, regulation and expression of sexual and aggressive impulses, formation of attachments to other individuals, organised initiation and completion of purposeful behaviour, and the inhibition of irrelevant and inappropriate behaviour.

(Grigsby and Schneiders, 1991, pp. 23–9)

The evolution of survival-related functions depends on the capacity for accurate multi-level memory. Indeed, if humans were incapable of storing, and retrieving accurate, detailed memories of a perceived life threat, survival beyond a few generations would be unlikely. Although we must be capable of "dissociating" various kinds of knowledge from our conscious awareness to develop the capacity for abstract, symbolic thinking, survival would be impossible if we were incapable of remembering our daily, necessary life-sustaining functions.

Evolved memory capacities

Humans have evolved complex methods of perceiving, assimilating and accommodating to change in ways that enhance the survival potential of individuals as well as the species. Inherent conflicts can arise between the dual, innate evolutionary goals – survival of the individual and survival of the species – which co-exist but are not identical. Individuals perceive and respond to the environment in diverse ways related to the effects of genetic endowment and environmental factors on the developing organism. It is this very diversity that permits our species to survive under changing conditions. Ironically, however, this particular "species-protecting" mechanism may not foster the survival of every individual, as individuals who respond in a rigid, specific, but life-preserving, way to potential threats in the initial environment may not be well adapted to the eventual changes in the environment. Consider what happens to a population when the environment is perceived as unpredictable and unsafe: innate physiological responses to the perception of threat compel individuals to act in self-protective ways (to enhance personal survival). In such an unknown or unpredictable environment, they may be forced to act "without knowing", an experience that is often accompanied by a state of anxiety. In chronic or extreme situations, this anxiety may intensify into a state of alarm, panic or terror (Janoff-Bulman, 1992; Marris, 1974).

The neurologically based alarm state involves certain changes in the blood flow, electrical potential and intensity of activity in various regions of the brain. The physiological and psychological changes that occur in alarmed or frightened individuals have been well documented (Conway, 1994; Schore, 1994; van der Kolk, 1987). Pervasive, measurable consequences of such changes in the quality and type of brain function include alterations in the cognitive capacity, perceptual experiences, affective intensity and responsivity of the alarmed individual (Frewen & Lanius, 2006; Grigsby & Stevens, 2000; Lanius et al., 2004; Udwin, 1993). When an unpredictable, changing environment persists, individuals begin to function in a chronic state of physiological and mental alarm. This alteration in normal functioning produces measurable changes in brain development (Edelman, 1987; Grigsby & Schneiders, 1991; Grigsby et al., 1991; Schore, 2002, 2003) and predictable behavioural sequelae (Herman, 1992; Perry, 2009; Perry et al., 1995; Udwin, 1993; Udwin & Dennis, 1995).

Importantly, the degree of external stimulation required to trigger an alarm state varies across individuals. Once the alarm–fear–terror continuum is triggered, physiological survival needs take precedence over psychological needs as innate self-survival responses are activated. This hierarchical response to the environment normally ensures that humans do not become so distracted by the "inner" world that they endanger their lives in the "real" world of physical needs and vulnerabilities.

What has all this to do with the "memory debate" of the late 20th and early 21st centuries? Perhaps, a great deal. In fact, the best indication that the "memory debate" has become related to our sense of survival is the fact that the academic discussions of human memory capacity frequently escalate to a level of affective intensity normally triggered only when one believes one's "life is under threat". How can we understand our defence of certain conceptualisations of the accuracy and fallibility of human memory as though our lives depended on the outcome?

I believe that more than professional identity is at stake here. A crucial feature of our understanding of the world in which we live is our knowledge of ourselves. If we know our history, our capacity to function in certain situations, and our potential for resolving conflicts or crises in our lives, we have a certain level of confidence about dealing with the future. When we are uncertain whether we know our own history, we are rendered unable to predict our responses to unexpected or threatening events; we fear we will be left exposed to extreme danger. Both psychological and physical threats then act as triggers for survival-related defences. Learned helplessness (Seligman, 1975) and chronic unresolved mourning (Marris, 1974; Murray-Parkes & Stevenson-Hinde, 1982) are commonly seen in individuals and cultures where an experience of unavoidable traumatic loss has transformed a learned, ad hoc response ("state") into a stable filter for experiencing the world (a "trait") (Perry et al., 1995) in which there is "no way" to stop the pain, predict the future, or resolve conflicts. The normal assumptions made by members of a society – that the world is predictable and basically safe, that we can be agents operating on our own behalf, that we are capable of making positive changes in our environment – are shattered by experiences of unavoidable, life-threatening catastrophe (Janoff-Bulman, 1992). In a rapidly changing, often alarming environment, such as that of the last three decades, the mere acceptance of the possibility that (as clinicians are telling us) experience-based aspects of human memory may be held totally out of awareness – completely unavailable to conscious verbal or visual image recall but able to exert a powerful, controlling impact on our behaviours and interactions with others – can trigger uncertainty, anxiety, and, eventually, fear. The knowledge that we may not know our capacities, our histories or ourselves tacitly undermines our sense of security by calling into question our competence to deal with the uncertainties of our future.

Selective exclusion: a normal defence against "knowing"

Bowlby (1985, 1988) described the ways in which, when faced with a personal/environmental crisis, human minds can defensively engage in a type of perceptual blocking that allows the continued existence of a secure framework for understanding and a feeling security in the environment and one's felt experience. This capability reduces the sense of confusion or alarm we experience when confronted with information that, if taken in, would threaten our established sense of ourselves. He describes "selective exclusion" – a process that affects all aspects of our perceptual and cognitive functions, from the receiving of sensory perceptions to the storing and retrieval of vital, related information regarding a specific situation. Bowlby states that,

> throughout a person's life he is engaged in excluding, or shutting out, a large proportion of all the information that is reaching him; secondly, that he does so only after its relevance to himself has been assessed; and thirdly that this process of selective exclusion is usually carried out without his being in any way aware of its happening.
>
> (1985, p. 193)

Once it is "selectively excluded", knowledge can remain inaccessible to conscious recall for many years, only to be "remembered" when suddenly triggered by something in a later environment, or when the knowledge no longer threatens the security of the individual.

Although current neuropsychological research substantiates the human capacity for selective exclusion (Williams, 1992), the concept was seminal when first proposed by Bowlby (Hamilton, 1985). Theories developed prior to the 1980s were generally limited to singular cause-and-effect formulations of human development. Experiments were designed to discover "the hidden cause" of symptoms (effects) that eluded comprehension. Specific efforts were made to isolate the human function under investigation to "eliminate any distortion or influence" resulting from any other source. Importantly, the computer – which can be used to simulate and to analyse massive amounts of information that simultaneously originate from many sources – was not yet in use in biological research.

With the development of complex, multiple-processor computers, a vastly enhanced capacity for information gathering and analysis became available. New technology introduced the possibility of observing and recording dynamic processes in human development. Since the mid-1970s, Magnetic Resonance Imaging (MRI), Positron Electron Tomography (PET), and ultrasound procedures have provided the means for the relatively non-intrusive monitoring of the physiological functions of living individuals in the service of medical and developmental research. In terms of understanding brain function, the combination of the abilities – first to monitor multi-level physiological changes and then to computer-analyse and model the complex, interactive processes – has enabled us to glimpse the formerly unimaginable, dynamic complexity of normal human thought and perceptual processes. Researchers and clinicians have worked in the last 25 years to create a language and a model for understanding the nonlinear complexity of human brain functions (Gaensbauer, 2016; Gaensbauer et al., 1995; Grigsby & Hartlaub, 1994; Grigsby & Stevens, 2002; Skarda & Freeman, 1987). It is to this framework that we must turn to integrate knowledge of interactive processes into a conceptual framework that clarifies and corrects the unavoidable distortions and inaccuracies of our previous one-dimensional, purposefully limited models of scientific experimental "accuracy".

Memory: conscious and non-conscious / declarative and non-declarative

We are developing an increasingly complex understanding of the multiple capacities for representation in human memory: case material from patients with documented traumatic histories (Herman, 1993; Sinason, 1994) is supported by neurocognitive research findings describing a multi-modular brain system that includes a complex memory capacity in which verbal (declarative) knowledge and non-verbalisable (non-declarative or procedural) knowledge can be consciously associated or non-consciously selectively excluded and dissociated from conscious memory (Grigsby 1991a, 1991b; Mishkin, 1992; Sinason, 2002).

In his review of the literature on declarative and non-declarative memory systems, Squire (1992) offered the following definitions: "Declarative (or explicit) memory refers to memory for words, scenes, faces and stories. It is assessed by conventional tests of recall and recognition. It is a memory for facts and events" (p. 232). "It can be brought to mind and content can be declared" (Cohen, 1984; Cohen & Squire, 1980). By contrast, non-declarative (including procedural and implicit) memory is utilised in "non-conscious" processes. This type of knowledge is grouped within several subsystems in the brain – the subgroups having in common only the fact that the memories cannot be consciously accessed, recalled, and verbalised. Examples of "non-declarative" learning are (1) the knowledge acquired during skill learning: motor skills and perceptual and cognitive skills, (2) habit formation and (3) emotional learning or classical conditioning. In other words, this knowledge is expressed through performance rather than recollection (Squire, 1992, p. 233).

"Procedural" memory is one type of non-declarative memory; it records habit-forming and skill-learning experiences but is often not accessible to verbal recall. In many instances, however, procedural and declarative (verbalisable) memory are linked; for example, knowing that you know how to play checkers, and being able to tell someone else how to play, is declarative knowledge. Understanding the physical interactive patterns and actually moving the pieces rests on consciously associated procedural knowledge. By contrast, under various circumstances, declarative and non-declarative (procedural) memories of a certain traumatic experience may become completely dissociated (Cohen & Squire, 1980; Emde et al., 1991; Grigsby & Hartlaub, 1994; Teicher, 2002).

A key feature of the various, non-conscious mental processes involves the ability of non-declarative memory to "support long-lasting changes in performance following a single encounter" (Squire, 1992). A single near-death experience, such as a near-drowning or a serious auto accident, can alter an individual's sense of self and behaviour for years – irrespective of whether it is accessible to declarative memory. In most cases, the memory of the event will be part of one's procedural, non-declarative memory for a lifetime (Terr, 1994).

Procedural and declarative memory in human figure drawings

There is evidence that procedural memory is fully functional even in early infancy, before the development of language (Brandt, 2011; Hartman & Burgess, 1993; Schore, 2001; Tulving, 1987). A child of 4 or 5 years without conscious memory of a traumatic, life-threatening experience in the first year of life can accurately recreate the dynamic situation in play (Gaensbauer, 2002). A tendency to re-enact (Terr, 1990) or portray in drawings (Burgess & Hartman, 1993; Moore, 1994b; Wohl & Kaufman, 1985) some aspects of both consciously remembered and unconscious early traumatic experiences is well documented in research regarding post-traumatic responses in children (Perry, 1997; Pynoos & Eth, 1986; Pynoos, Steinberg & Wraith, 1994). Traumatic experiences – whether related to illness, abuse, or other events – can be held in declarative memory, and these memories can be recalled and verbalised as well as represented in drawings (Coates & Moore, 1997; Goodwin, 1982; Wohl & Kaufman, 1985). In some cases, however, the interactive process or body memories of traumatic experience will be held in non-declarative memory – in procedural form – while any declarative memory of what occurred is dissociated. This dissociation of procedural and declarative memory may occur when an event involves intense traumatic affect, or when the individual was an infant or child at the time of the trauma (Moore, 1994a, 1994b). These non-declarative, procedural memories cannot be articulated verbally but will be evidenced in behaviour in specific ways, such as in habit formation.

A child's drawing process, as well as the drawing itself, may reflect specific non-declarative, procedural memories of early childhood trauma (Coates & Moore, 1997; Moore, 1994b, 1995). This has obvious relevance to human personality organisation, conscious and unconscious self-perception, and the levels of self-knowledge reflected in drawings. With careful study, we are increasing our understanding of the potential levels of representation in a drawing (Coates & Moore, 1997; Moore, 1990, 1994a, 1994b), realising that both lived experience (i.e. procedural knowledge) and constructed meaning (including defences and coping strategies) are potentially expressed in drawings; this allows the psychotherapist to gain a deeper comprehension of the child's lived experience and to limit cognitive questions and interpretive comments appropriately. Operating from this perspective, the therapist recognises that non-symbolic representations may reflect memories that cannot be verbalised at the time the drawing is created (Gaensbauer et al., 1995; Moore, 1995). However, one can always be certain that a drawing includes many levels of meaning, reflective of knowledge held in multi-modular memory systems – some of which can be made conscious, and some of which are dissociated from conscious, verbalisable thought.

Human evolution, complex brain process, in the on-going memory debate

Multi-modular memory categories differ so greatly that it might be considered misleading to refer to them all using the same terminology: i.e. "memories". In fact, the human brain has evolved – precisely for reasons of adaptiveness in a changing and potentially dangerous environment – diverse methods of perceiving and storing both declarative and procedural experience, not surprisingly, in different regions of the brain. Brain scan/computer-facilitated techniques, such as PET and MRI, now allow researchers to observe brain processes in awake and active subjects. A recent study found that different individuals showed distinct variations in their brain activation patterns while considering the identical problem. As all subjects arrived at the same correct answer, this important individual diversity in process would not have been recognised had the highly divergent patterns of brain activity during problem-solving not been monitored with imaging technology, this important individual diversity in the process would not have been recognised (Gur, Mozley & Mozley, 1995).

Gender differences in the brain functions involved in information processing were also revealed in Gur's research. The complex influence of hormones not only on brain development (from foetal states to adult years) but on the brain processes recruited on an immediate task-by-task, day-by-day basis can be observed and measured. Gender analyses of these data demonstrate that males and females generally activated different areas of the brain when answering a specific question, again, despite the fact that all reached the correct answer (Gur et al., 1987; Gur et al., 1995). This diversity in problem-solving reflects the complementarity of gender and individual differences and argues against there being a "best" way to process information, or a "superior" way in which to come to a decision. As the context is part of the function – rather than separate from it – divergent potential responses are more adaptive given the variety of potential contexts. Technology that enables simultaneous assessment of brain processes and the environment has produced the revolutionary understanding that physiological process and environment are an interactive whole that irreducibly constitutes a given function.

It is no longer possible to use a single aspect of the process to determine "what memory is". The context within which we gather our "data" regarding memory as well as the context in which such memories are initially formed is part of the function of memory (Grigsby & Schneiders, 1991; Grigsby et al., 1991). If we do not know who the subject is – what an individual's early experience has been, what his or her constitutional (genetic) givens are, what the presented stimuli mean to the research subject – we can determine only a minute fraction of the given brain function we seek to understand. Under these conditions, we may use "answers" that are not only limited in applicability but are also distorted and inaccurate as a basis for broader conclusions. Attempts to identify the limits of "human memory capacity" are severely constrained precisely by the specific methods chosen to "measure" memory and by the exact language used to elicit recall. Experiments performed with volunteer subjects who are asked to remember nonsense syllables in a laboratory setting offer some information about what can be recalled by a select group of subjects under specific laboratory conditions.

The group results of these "cognitive memory capacity" studies can't help us anticipate or evaluate what parts, if any, of a previous traumatic experience a particular individual can recall and articulate, as the context and quality of memory activated vary dramatically. In addition, when one individual is asked – in separate environments, at different times, or in different emotional states – to recount the details of a specific event, he or she may recall slightly different material in each instance; this is precisely because the context within which memories are retrieved allows or prevents access to some parts of the memory itself (Briere, Scott & Weathers, 2005; Courtois, 2008; Grigsby et al., 1991; Sgroi, 1981). Perhaps our previous inability to differentiate and identify these unique memory functions – each of which is an irreducible whole comprised of both physiological and psychological processes and environmental context – has also fuelled the intensity of the conflict in the current debate.

Complications in the study of memory in the late 20th and early 21st centuries

Having been carefully taught to ask questions that clarify complex issues by isolating one concept from another, we must now learn to avoid asking exactly those unanswerable questions: e.g. "how reliable is memory"? It is now abundantly clear that there is no single correct answer. The context, the precursors, the internal motivation of the experimental subject, the affective state of the individual at the time of the event and the time of recall, all influence performance on memory tasks in everyday situations as well as in the laboratory. However, evolutionary theory makes it clear that if all memories were stored as "inaccurate distortions of reality", the dual goals of survival – of the individual and of the species – would be violated (Bowlby, 1969, 1973, 1980, 1985).

In addition, there are errors inherent in generalising from the results of controlled laboratory experiments on cognitive memory to judgements of capacity in real-life situations. When bridging the gap between research and clinical practice, we must always remember that using results from studies comparing responses from many subjects (as a group) to evaluate an individual or a specific patient's responses is always inappropriate. Research results generally compare the most common characteristics of one group with the most common characteristics of another group. In most cases, however, a number of individuals within each population will have some characteristics that are unlike or dissimilar to those of the majority. The diversity of these individuals' characteristics (or symptoms) does not necessarily deny that person group membership; they simply do not show identical characteristics common to the majority of members. Equally, an individual patient's symptoms that show a similarity to – or dissimilarity from – those of a group profile only predict group membership; they do not guarantee it.

Applying laboratory based cognitive memory research results to a single clinical case is no guarantee of the accuracy of the assessment of memory function. Our capacity to observe and analyse various brain functions as dynamic processes is expanding at an incredible rate. We must assimilate new data into our "body of knowledge" on the subject of memory at a rate that often exceeds our ability to integrate it into existing frameworks. This highly stressful, rapidly changing environment for learning may be related to the continued trend in memory research to revert to simple, single cause-and-effect studies, seeking "the answer", asking single-focus measurement questions to elicit a "correct" answer regarding the "reliability of human memory for early events".

The need to know is an aspect of human functioning that underlies many survival instincts; however, we need to be able to predict not only our own capacity to recognise danger and respond effectively to crises or life events but also to anticipate what the environment will be like. "Not knowing" triggers a state of anxiety. In times of great stress or threat, we make decisions of a dichotomous nature, usually related to taking one action or another. Consciously deciding what we "know to be true" allows us to experience greater psychological clarity about the presence of potential threat in our environment. A sense of "knowing" our environment produces a calmer inner state of mind – less physically aroused and hypervigilant to external threat (innate self-survival capacities associated with the mid-brain and brainstem), more able to concentrate on thought and planning strategies (self- and species-specific survival capacities developed using prefrontal lobes and the cortex). A reactive, polarised type of decision making may be – often is – appropriate in life-or-death emergency situations; however, it is not appropriate when new theories and information are being presented and need to be critically considered in light of extant knowledge.

Anxiety eliciting conditions are not conducive to careful, deliberative, integrative and abstract thinking. We, the authors within this book, are as caught within our historical frame as were previous authors; as we respond from our embeddedness in our current historical context, our thinking is likely to be unconsciously influenced by the exact elements we are trying to articulate and understand. New information about human memory does not fit into the old theories, but our current chaotic, unpredictable environment may be a contributor to an increased sense of vulnerability that runs counter to the adaptive in-depth consideration necessary to deconstruct old frameworks to incorporate new knowledge. We may feel the urge to cling to what we have known as a way to survive and stabilise the turmoil of our current global, national, and local – political, social, economic – environments. By holding in mind the reality that our context is an inseparable aspect of who we are and what we are capable of knowing, we might allow ourselves to take a contemplative step back and seek thoughtful ways to counter the more unproductive, non-conscious, survival-related and thus, uncompromising, absolute responses that have fuelled much of the destructive polarisation and intense anger reflected in the decades-long "Memory Debate".

References

Bowlby, J. (1969). *Attachment and Loss: Attachment (Vol. 1: Attachment)*. London: The Hogarth Press and The Institute of Psycho-Analysis.

Bowlby, J. (1973). *Attachment and Loss: Separation (Vol. 2. Separation: Anxiety and Anger)*. London: The Hogarth Press and The Institute of Psycho-Analysis.

Bowlby, J. (1980). *Attachment and Loss: Loss (Vol. 3)*. London: The Hogarth Press and the Institute of Psycho-Analysis.

Bowlby, J. (1985). The role of childhood experience in cognitive disturbance. In M. M. A. Freeman (Ed.), *Cognition and Psychotherapy*. New York: Plenum Publishing, pp. 181–200.

Brandt, K., Perry, B., Seligman, S., Tronick, E. (2011). Infants' Meaning-Making and the Development of Mental Health Problems. *American Psychologist*, 66 (2), 107–119.

Briere, J., Scott, C., & Weathers, F. W. (2005). Peritraumatic and Persistent Dissociation in the Presumed Etiology of PTSD. *American Journal of Psychiatry*, 162, 2295–2301.

Burgess, A. & Hartman, C. (1993). Children's Drawings. *Child Abuse and Neglect*, 17, 161–168.

Coates, S. W. & Moore, M. S. (1997). The Complexity of Early Trauma: Representation and Transformation. *Psychoanalytic Inquiry*, 17, 286–311.

Cohen, N. J. (1984). Preserved learning Capacity in Amnesia: Evidence for Multiple Memory Systems. In L. R. Squire & N. Butters (Eds.), *Neuropsychology of Memory*. New York: Gilford Press, pp. 83–103.

Cohen, N. J. & Squire, L. R. (1980). Preserved Learning and Retention of Pattern-Analyzing Skill in Amnesia: Dissociation of Knowing How and Knowing That. *Science*, 210, 207–209.

Conway, A.V. (1994). Trance-Formations of Abuse. In V. Sinason (Ed.), *Treating Survivors of Satanist Abuse*. London: Routledge.

Courtois, C. (2008). Complex Trauma, Complex Reactions: Assessment and Treatment. *Psychological Trauma Theory Research Practice and Policy*doi:10.1037/1942–9681.S.1.86

Edelman, G. M. (1987). *Neural Darwinism: Theory of Neuronal Group Selection*. New York: Basic Books.

Emde, R., Biringen, Z., Clyman, R. & Oppenheim, D. (1991). The Moral Self of Infancy: Affective Core and Procedural Knowledge. *Developmental Review*, 11, 251–270.

Frewen, P. A. & Lanius, R.A. (2006). Neurobiology of Dissociation: Unity and Disunity in Mind–Body–Brain. *Psychiatric Clinics of North America*, 29, 113–128.

Gaensbauer, T. (2002). Representations of Trauma in Infancy: Clinical and Theoretical Implications for the Understanding of Early Memory. *Infant Mental Health Journal*, 23 (3), 259–277.

Gaensbauer, T. (2016). Moments of Meeting: The Relevance of Lou Sander's and Dan Stern's Conceptual Framework for Understanding the Development of Pathological Social Relatedness. *Infant Mental Health Journal*, 37 (2), 172–188.

Gaensbauer, T., Chatoor, I., Drell, M., Siegel, D. & Zeanah, C. H. (1995). Tramatic Loss in a One-Year-Old Girl. *Journal of the American Academy of Child & Adolescent Psychiatry*, 34 (4), 520–528.

Goodwin, J. (1982). Use of Drawings in Evaluating Children Who May Be Incest Victims. *Children and Youth Services Review*, 4, 269–278.

Grigsby, J. & Hartlaub, G. (1994). Procedural Learning and the Development and Stability of Character. *Perceptual and Motor Skills*, 79, 355–370.

Grigsby, J. & Schneiders, J. (1991). Neuroscience, Modularity and Personality Theory: Conceptual Foundations of a Model of Complex Human Functioning. *Psychiatry*, 54, 21–38.

Grigsby, J., Schneiders, J. & Kaye, K. (1991). Reality Testing, the Self and the Brain as Modular Distributed Systems. *Psychiatry*, 54, 39–54.

Grigsby, J. & Stevens, D. (2000). *The Neurodynamics of Personality*. New York: Guilford Press, p. 16.

Grigsby, J. & Stevens, D. (2002). Memory, Neurodynamics, and Human Relationships. *Psychiatry*, 65 (1), 13–34.

Gur, R. C., Gur, R. E., Obrist, W. D., Skolnick, B. E. & Reivich, M. (1987). Age and Regional Cerebral Blood Flow at Rest and During Cognitive Activity. *Archives of General Psychiatry*, 44, 617–621.

Gur, R. C., Mozley, L. H. & Mozley, P. D. (1995). Sex Differences in Regional Cerebral Glucose Metabolism During a Resting State. *Science*, 267, 528–531.

Hartman, C. & Burgess, A. W. (1993). Information Processing in Trauma. *Child Abuse and Neglect*, 17, 47–58.

Herman, J. (1992). *Trauma and Recovery*. New York: Basic Books.

Herman, J. (1993). Sequelae of Prolonged and Repeated Trauma: Evidence for a Complex Posttraumatic Syndrome (DESNOS). In J. R. T. Davidson & E. Foa (Eds.), *Post-traumatic Stress Disorder: DSM III and Beyond*. Washington, DC: American Psychiatric Press.

Janoff-Bulman, R. (1992). *Shattered Assumptions: Towards a New Psychology of Trauma*. New York: Free Press.

Lanius, R., Williamson, P. C., Densmore, M., Boksman, K., Neufeld, R. W., Gati, J. S. & Menon, R. S. (2004). The Nature of Traumatic Memories: A 4-T FMRI Functional Connectivity Analysis. *American Journal of Psychiatry*, 161 (1), 36–44.

Marris, P. (1974). *Loss and Change*. London: Routledge.

Moore, M. S. (1994a). Common Characteristics in the Drawings of Ritually Abused Children and Adults. In V. Sinason (Ed.), *Treating Survivors of Satanic Ritual Abuse*. London: Routledge, pp. 221–241.

Moore, M. S. (1994b). Reflections of Self: The Use of Drawings in Evaluating and Treating Physically Ill Children. In A. Erskine & D. Judd (Eds.), *The Imaginative Body: Treating Physically Ill Patients in Psychotherapy.* London: Whurr Publications.

Moore, M. S. (1995). *Complexity of Infant Trauma: Representation and Transformation.* Paper presented at the Australian Association of Infant Mental Health – Annual National Conference, Melbourne, Victoria, Australia.

Murray-Parkes, C. & Stevenson-Hinde, J. (Eds.). (1982). *The Place of Attachment in Human Behavior.* New York: Basic Books.

Perry, B. D. (1997). Incubated in Terror: Neurodevelopmental Factors in the "Cycle of Violence". In J. Osofsky (Ed.), *Children in a Violent Society.* New York: Guilford Press, pp. 124–149.

Perry, B. D. (2009). Examining Child Maltreatment Through a Neurodevelopmental Lens: Clinical Applications of the Neurosequential Model of Therapeutics (NMT). *Journal of Loss and Trauma,* 14, 240–255.

Perry, B. D., Pollard, R., Blakley, T., Baker, W. & Vigilante, D. (1995). Childhood Trauma, the Neurobiology of Adaptation and Use-Dependent Development of the Brain: How "states" become "traits". *Infant Mental Health Journal,* 16 (4), 271–291.

Pynoos, R. & Eth, S. (1986). Witness to Violence: the Child Interview. *Journal of the American Academy of Child & Adolescent Psychiatry,* 25 (3), 306–319.

Pynoos, R., Steinberg, A., & Wraith, R. (1994). A developmental Model of Childhood Traumatic Stress. In D. Cicchetti & D. Cohen (Eds.), *Manual of Developmental Psychopathology.* New York: J. Wiley & Sons.

Schore, A. N. (1994). *Affect Regulation and the Origin of the Self: The Neurobiology of Emotional Development.* New Jersey: Erlbaum.

Schore, A. N. (2001). The Effects of Early Relational Trauma on Right Brain Development, Affect Regulation, and Infant Mental Health Infant. *Mental Health Journal,* 22 (1–2), 201–269.

Schore, A. N. (2002). Advances in Neuropsychoanalysis, Attachment Theory, and Trauma Research: Implications for Self Psychology. *Psychoanalytic Dialogues,* 22, 433–484.

Schore, A. N. (2003). *Affect Dysregulation and Disorders of the Self.* New York: W.W. Norton.

Sgroi, S. (Ed.) (1981). *Handbook of Clinical Intervention in Child Sexual Abuse.* London: Free Press.

Sinason, V. (Ed.) (1994). *Treating Survivors of Satanist Abuse.* London/New York: Routledge.

Skarda, C. & Freeman, W. (1987). How Brains Make Chaos in Order To Make Sense of the World. *Behavioral and Brain Sciences,* 10, 161–195.

Teicher, M. H. (2002). Scars That Won't Heal: The Neurobiology of Child Abuse. *Scientific American,* 286, 68–75.

Tulving, E. (1987). Multiple Memory Systems and Consciousness. *Neurobiology,* 6, 67–80.

Udwin, O. (1993). Annotation: Children's Reactions to Traumatic Events. *J. of Child Psychology & Psychiatry,* 34 (2), 118–127.

Udwin, O. & Dennis, J. (1995). Psychological and behavioural phenotypes in geneti-
cally determined syndromes: a review of research findings. In G. O'Brien (Eds.),
Behavioural Phenotypes. London: Mac Keith Press, pp. 90–208.

Van der Kolk, B. A. (1987). *Psychological Trauma*. Washington, DC: American Psychiatric Press.

Williams, L. M. (1992). Adult Memories of Childhood Abuse. *Journal of the American
Professional Society on the Abuse of Children*, 5, 19–21.

Wohl, A. & Kaufman, B. (1985). *Silent Screams and Hidden Cries: A Compilation and
Interpretation of Artwork by Children from Violent Homes*. New York: Brunner
Mazel.

Chapter 12

What if I should die?

Jennifer Johns

In this chapter, Jennifer Johns describes the terrible physical countertransference impact on an analyst listening to a patient talk of systemic savage abuse in childhood. This raises the complex issue of truth in the consulting-room.

A psychoanalyst, not young or inexperienced and to the best of her knowledge in perfect health, was sitting very still and listening to an extremely distressed patient speaking with great difficulty, of memories implying savage, perverse and systematic many-layered cruelty in childhood.

During the story, the analyst suddenly developed pain in her own chest. The pain was central, and gradually became severe enough to make her seriously anxious about herself and to prevent her ordinary concentration on what was happening in the session. She began to try to recollect old fragments of her training in medicine as the pain spread upwards into her jaw, and she became more and more frightened that she was having a heart attack. She tried to reassure herself that the pain, though acute, was not typically cardiac, and intellectually she tried to make sense of it in the naive hope that, once made sense of, it would go away. Unable to listen to or concentrate on her patient, she told herself that it was probably indigestion, or not in fact real, and chided herself for failing her patient at such a vital moment. She told herself that she must pull herself together and return to her concentration on the patient and the session, and that until the pain went down her left arm, she would not interrupt the session. However, she was very frightened.

On another level, the analyst's mental conflict was acute too, since even in the midst of the fear and pain she recognised that what she had been hearing, and had stopped being able to hear, was a story carrying the implication of the most barbaric human behaviour – the most horrifying that she had heard in 20 years of analytic practice – and she found herself beginning to doubt her own ego-strength when discovering the inability to listen to it and to realise that it was possible that, in putting her through this physical ordeal, her body was refusing to allow her to submit herself to the psychological one of taking in what her patient was saying. It was not the first time that the story had been told, but on each occasion further details of dehumanising and debasing perversity emerged, and the patient had needed time and space to be able to reach the thoughts about them.

DOI: 10.4324/9781003193159-13

There are, of course, occasions when listening to a patient that an analyst (and the analyst was, of course, myself) may quite consciously feel a wish not to hear, a wish to keep some memory, thought, or fantasy out of the mind, and afterwards a knowledge that what one has just heard about is something that, given the choice, one would rather not have known, thoughts that cannot be unthought, memories that cannot be unremembered, words that must always leave a trace, ineradicable evidence of the most deliberately cruel and perverse elements of human life. An analyst, however, in offering a mind to others, to receive their thoughts and memories and fantasies, must therefore have some optimism about his or her own mental strength and capacity to survive such onslaughts, especially when trying to help those who have not psychologically survived. In my turmoil, I accused myself of arrogance, of having held a naive presumption that in my professional life I could take anything, manage any material that my patient might give me. I felt that I was facing, as well as the reality of failing my patient so badly, the humiliation of failing my own egoideal, and, as well as the shocks associated with what I had heard and was being asked to believe, I was shocked at how badly my own body was letting me down.

All psychoanalysts are used to the everyday analytic task of the examination of their own inner world alongside that of their patients, the examination of their own thoughts and feelings, and the everlasting and recurrent psychoanalytic question as to the relationship between their own inner world and that of their patients, the conscious and unconscious influences of each upon the other. The term countertransference is understood as something rather different and complementary – the influence, frequently unconsciously experienced, of the patient's transference to the analyst upon the analyst. The analyst knows to watch for countertransferences, in so far as that is possible during analytic sessions, countertransference being so largely unconscious, sometimes so unconscious that its existence may be manifested by bodily sensations, and analysts are also used to the phenomenon of recognising with hindsight how their own countertransferences can affect a session – there are times when patients point that out directly and clearly, and times when it is possible to puzzle it out for oneself. There are also times when it is appropriate to share particularly obscure problems with a colleague; on this particular occasion, there were reasons why this had not, in fact, been possible. These situations were familiar, but what had happened on this day was a new phenomenon. I had never, so far as I could remember, experienced such an overwhelmingly painful and frightening bodily response to a patient, or felt so terrifyingly helpless and in real and imminent danger of death. A certain common sense told me that it is not impossible to become ill in terms of physical reality, and that illness can strike at any time without necessarily being related to the patient, and warned me against a kind of magical thinking involving a denial of my own mortality, but I did not find this convincing – the immediacy of the physical response was too closely related to the patient's material to be, I felt, accidental.

In calmer moments, it is possible to recall that by means of what is called projective identification an analyst's internal state can reflect either the affects of the patient as the subject in the situation being remembered or dealt with, or the affects of the patient's object in that situation – and work with traumatised patients leads one to know that not only is terrible pain, fear and suffering traumatic, but so too is the utter helplessness of being a victim, and, moreover, that the further helplessness of being either unable to help another victim or of believing oneself in some way responsible for the other's suffering is cumulatively traumatic. These pieces of everyday professional knowledge were, however, unavailable in the acute moment. When I recovered, much later, it was possible to think out the occurrence more calmly and to realise that the helplessness, pain and fear felt might indeed have been related to the overwhelming experience that the patient had been describing, which had contained elements of all these. Surprised most of all by the bodily phenomenon, I later wondered whether the pain was due to my own oesophagus having gone into spasm as a physical attempt to defend myself against swallowing the patient's material. Swallowing would mean acceptance of it, and I recognised the very strong wish not to accept such evidence of human perverse cruelty. It may be important to state that although with this person there had been times earlier in the treatment when I had found myself questioning what I heard, I had in fact reached a stage when that intellectual barrier was past. My mind could picture all too well – but it made me feel very ill, and very frightened.

It is the job of a psychoanalyst to help the sufferer make sense of a frightening and confusing inner world, and, in order to do that, the analyst must be able to understand something of the fears and confusions of that inner world. Those fears and confusions are frequently, though not always, related to perceptions of the outer world, and those perceptions are, of course, received by a perceptual apparatus with a developmental history of its own. The perceptual apparatus itself may have been damaged and distorted during that development, even to the extent of being unable to perceive an event, or the memory of an event, in the same way that another, less distorted person might. When an analyst listens to a patient speaking about unbearable pain or communicating it by non-verbal or even unconscious communication, as in projective identification, the analyst must hope that the experience will be bearable by himself or herself. That will mean containing the experience, processing it, and eventually being able, with the patient, to put it into words in such a way that the patient can accept it.

What happens when the flood of feeling from the patient makes the analyst unable to think or contain the experience? This may be sharing the patient's historical state of having been overwhelmed, but it is of no use at all in making sense of it. It would be easy to say, and perhaps true, that I, the analyst in question, was myself inadequately analysed, that had I known myself better I might have been more able to contain the situation of horror presented to me. However, the catalogue of human cruelty is very long, and, while one may be prepared for many of its entries, particularly those based on intimate two-body relationships or even the kind of institutionalised torture of a concentration camp, each of which can have its own bizarre rationality, the organised distortion of reason that is entered under the label "evil" is different. Systematic perversion of all values, which overturns all expectation of predictable response in favour of the savage joy of perversity – by which I mean annihilation of all that is good, for the sake of that destruction only – is painful and difficult to hear. Those who habitually work with such material agree on the need for colleague support and limitation of exposure to it, to protect themselves. It is also important that any colleagues consulted to help deal with and accept these things have experience of having tried themselves to help similar distress, so that the initial barrier of acceptance of the horror of the extremes of human cruelty is passed.

It seems that very young infants already need to make sense of the happenings in themselves and their environment by means of creating a narrative for themselves, as a way of making some sort of order or sense of the phenomena observed and experienced, and this would seem to be related to the beginning of the epistemophilic drive to understand, to find out, to master confusion by knowing. Perhaps those who find the world most confusing develop into the most insistently curious, if they are not too daunted by their confusion or inhibited by the environment's response to it. The question of when, and to what degree, curiosity and the need to establish mental order and a narrative (or, when older, a search for an actual explanation of confusing data) may be defensive against too-frightening confusion is an interesting one. The need to know, the need to establish so-called historical truth, may be a defence against overwhelming affect. Amongst our other defences when we feel utterly helpless, we may take refuge in an attempt at mental mastery, so that even in suffering pain or defeat we are comforted in that we can at least understand the mind of the person who caused it. This creates the kind of situation in which an about-to-be executed victim forgives his torturers in another version of "Father, forgive them …"

Among the attempts at self-preservation there is a wish in human beings – and this includes those who become analysts – to establish, or be able to establish, the veridicality of new information. In an analyst, this may be defensive, for a search for "facts" can allow distance from the reality of the psychic pain of the sufferer. It may feel much safer to escape into the outside world where "facts" are felt to be verifiable, solid matters. However, such an escape is a betrayal of the analytic task, which is to understand the inner world of the patient, especially *in extremis*. For those in contact with the world that requires facts, the legal or protective world, this can be a nightmare – one aspect of their professional world needs something called proof, another needs understanding of inner pain, and the two may be antithetical.

For myself, there is no way that the experience of having suffered the fear for my very life that occurred with my patient could in any way be called to account as legal proof of anything. I am safe from that requirement. I am left with an enormous question – to what extent was my own terrifying experience in any way validating of my patient's inner world? My answer to that question is that it is. It was important that my understanding of the inner position should happen.

It seemed to me that my very body answered my patient. I did not want to know the extent of the experience – and the patient had been very sparing of detail, very careful to dose my exposure to it – and I believe that in the end my body tried to refuse it.

What happened next? My patient, in fact, noticed my distress and ended the session early, also distressed at the effect on me. For many later sessions, the effect was discussed and the fear of causing my death became paramount. The quality of work altered, and the elaboration of the story was delayed. The patient retreated into a different way of working, and the issue, for the moment, changed. I regretted my failure, though I could not have avoided it, and the question of the repetition of past failures came into prominence.

Though this very frightening experience has never, I am glad to say, been repeated, I do class it as a manifestation of bodily countertransference, as a communication from my patient of the extreme overwhelming by fear of death, guilt and horror.

The question of veridicality, of the search for so-called historical truth, is a matter for lawyers and the police. Analysts must know that when a patient brings material of great anguish, the analyst is hearing a true story of anguish.

Chapter 13

Finding a new narrative

Meaningful responses to "false memory" disinformation

Michael Salter

The success of "false memory syndrome" advocacy during the 1990s was largely due to its compelling narrative features. Scientific evidence relevant to traumatic memory remains critical to the development of effective therapy and successful abuse investigations and prosecutions. However, this chapter also encourages practitioners and advocates to develop public narratives about trauma and abuse that are not only accurate but solutions-focused and hopeful.

Introduction

> You cannot take someone's story away without giving them a new one. It is not enough to challenge an old narrative, however outdated and discredited it may be. Change happens only when you replace it with another. When we develop the right story, and learn how to tell it, it will infect the minds of people across the political spectrum. Those who tell the stories run the world.
>
> (Monbiot, 2017, p. 1)

In the 1980s, journalists around the world began telling a new story about child sexual abuse. Beginning in the United States, and followed by Europe and Australia, the media climate changed dramatically from disinterest to widespread, high-profile coverage. Child abuse was, according to the news, a "hidden epidemic" of extraordinary proportions (Beckett, 1996). Only ten years later, the media position on abuse had undergone an almost complete inversion. By the early 1990s, the new "hidden epidemic" was not widespread abuse, but "false memories" of abuse, encouraged by collective neurosis and the malfeasance of therapists and social workers (Kitzinger, 2004). In response, mental health professionals, abuse survivors and their advocates presented research data on abuse, trauma and memory, and sought to clarify misrepresentations and misunderstandings about therapeutic practice. While these efforts were laudable, they failed to dislodge the "false memory" story from its hegemonic position in the mass media and public imagination. Accurate information, alone, could not compete with the emotional appeals of "false memory" advocates.

DOI: 10.4324/9781003193159-14

This chapter draws from George Monbiot's (2017) thoughts on the political power of storytelling. He emphasises that stories function as schema through which people organise information and develop a sense of order and purpose. It is a mistake, he warns, to try to rely on data to challenging a misleading story since "[t]he only thing that can displace a story is a story" (Monbiot, 2017, p. 3). In short, information is not sufficient to challenge disinformation: we must also supply a meaningful framework in which that information makes sense. In this chapter, I suggest that the success of "false memory" was due, largely, to its compelling narrative features. False memory advocates were skilled at retelling the story of child abuse as a drama with heroes (people falsely accused of abuse and their allies) and villains (therapists, social workers, feminists) locked in a battle of good (science, reason, rationality) against the forces of darkness (dogma, fantasy, hysteria). Attempts by experts in trauma and dissociation to counter this story with data have, at times, struggled for purchase, since they have not challenged the affective foundations of the "false memory" narrative.

In this chapter, I argue that we have the opportunity to tell a new, and more hopeful, story about abuse and trauma. While the "false memory" story persists, it has been destabilised by revelations of widespread clergy and institutional abuse, and its valorisation of staunch individualism and devaluing of health and welfare services has lost much of its sheen. At the same time, the conceptual apparatus of trauma has taken on increasing social and political as well as psychological significance as a descriptor for the violation of human relationality and the restorative power of care and support. Increased public interest and understanding of trauma provides much of the material for counter-narratives that oppose the alienating individualism and cynicism promoted by "false memory" advocates. As public and professional interest in trauma grows, "storifying" trauma in principled and solutions-focused ways offers a genuine alternative to the outmoded narratives of the past.

The meaning of abuse

The exponential increase in media coverage of child sexual abuse in the 1980s can leave the impression that sexual abuse was discovered only 40 years ago. In fact, historical scholarship shows that child sexual abuse has been the subject of sustained media interest and public anxiety throughout the modern period (Finnane & Smaal, 2016). However, while an incident of child sexual abuse might have been deplored, what child sexual abuse meant – what it signified or symbolised – was quite ambiguous prior to the 1980s. Notions of "sin" and moral degeneracy attributed blame and stigma to the child victim as well as the perpetrator. Pseudo-Freudian theories of childhood sexuality suggested that children fantasied about and desired sexual contact with adults (Shengold, 2000). Such arguments were recast as scientific truth from the 1950s within the libertarian milieu of the science of "sexology", where researchers such as Alfred Kinsey documented a high prevalence of child sexual abuse but suggested it was harmless or even beneficial

(Olafson, Corwin & Summit, 1993). In short, the social construction of child sexual abuse has been messy, incoherent and morally ambivalent.

Intersecting feminist and child protection concerns in the 1970s proposed a simpler and emotionally moving formulation: that child sexual abuse was common, harmful and the fault of the adult not the child. Feminist consciousness-raising evolved alongside improvements in paediatric expertise during the 1960s and the 1970s, generating new knowledge and evidence for the frequency and effects of child abuse. Changes to legislation and family law, including the advent of mandatory reporting legislation, drove an unprecedented increased in abuse reports and investigations in the 1980s. These new cases vividly illustrated claims of child abuse as a "hidden epidemic", resulting in mass media coverage of child sexual abuse as a significant, but suppressed, social problem from the early to late 1980s (Beckett, 1996). Abuse stories included multiple dramatic elements that enhanced their newsworthiness and public salience: sexual predators, innocent children, descriptions of sexual violence and suggestions of a widespread "conspiracy of silence". This formulation of child sexual abuse has remained a point of reference in the public imagination and political discourse ever since.

Conservatism, neoliberalism and the story of "false memories"

While mental health, child protection and law enforcement agencies grappled with an unprecedented number of sexual abuse cases, the political trend of the 1980s was towards *dis*investment in welfare and support agencies (Campbell, 2021). The defunding of social supports was legitimised by a partnership between social conservatives and economic neoliberals who shared, albeit for different reasons, a dislike for state intervention in private life, and a focus on the restoration of family privacy (Cooper, 2017). This political backdrop had two interlinked effects on responses to child abuse. The first was material. Child protection and health services found themselves tasked to respond to child sexual abuse as a major priority without an equivalent increase in funds or personnel. Indeed, in some cases, welfare and health budgets were *shrinking* even as agencies were faced with an increasing number and complexity of sexual abuse cases.

The second effect was discursive. In such a political climate, where state agencies were routinely characterised as incompetent and oppressive, difficulties in child abuse investigations were liable to be blamed on services and professionals rather than systemic problems, such as a lack of resources and personnel. Those accused of child abuse found a sympathetic hearing where they linked the allegations against them to state over-reach or incompetence (Hechler, 1988).

The inevitable result was described by Campbell (2021) in her analysis of the Cleveland case in England in the late 1980s, where a large number of children were removed from their families due to suspicion of sexual abuse. The local children's hospital and welfare services experienced an influx of vulnerable children in the midst of a resourcing crisis caused by budget cuts, triggering a systemic failure that was blamed on individual professionals. The case has become widely remembered in the United Kingdom as an example of "false allegations" encouraged by professional malpractice, despite significant evidence of sexual abuse amongst the group of children removed by social services (Campbell, 2021; Donaldson & O'Brien, 1995).

This pattern was evident throughout the Global North during the 1980s, as child protection and law enforcement were confronted with unexpectedly complex and severe allegations of abuse. A number of high-profile cases included allegations of multiple victims and multiple perpetrators, and descriptions of sadistic abuse, ritual abuse and the manufacture of child sexual abuse material (Salter, 2013). In the absence of adequate training, personnel or policy frameworks to facilitate interagency cooperation, these complex cases tested partnerships between child protection and law enforcement, who faced clashing professional cultures and competing imperatives in their work with children. These cases also highlighted the barriers faced by young and traumatised witnesses in the criminal justice system, with children subject to hostile cross-examination and forced to confront their alleged abuser/s directly in court. Difficulties in investigating or prosecuting these cases were highlighted by influential journalists as evidence of a rising tide of false abuse allegations, driven by zealous state agencies and the incompetence of feminised "caring" professions, such as therapy and social work (Cheit, 2014; Salter, 2018).

The media focus on "false allegations" only accelerated during the 1990s. As legislative changes in many US states enabled adults abused as children to pursue civil suits or criminal charges against their abusers, adults accused of abuse organised a counter-movement under the banner of "false memory syndrome" (Brown, Scheflin & Hammond, 1998). This "syndrome" described the development of false memories of childhood abuse by adults, often with the encouragement of a therapist. The "false memory" movement combined appeals to scientific authority with gripping stories of happy families torn apart by therapists who supposedly manipulated clients into "recovering memories" of incest that never took place. "False memory" advocacy proved to be extraordinarily successful in influencing the media debate, with journalists amongst the most vocal champions of the "false memory" position (Kitzinger, 2004). According to the mass media, the threat to public safety was no longer men who abused children, but rather those professionals who purported to respond to child abuse and its effects. Therapists and child protection workers, in particular, were characterised as obsessed, incompetent and perverse in their focus on abuse.

Campbell (2003) argues that the "false memory" narrative was grounded in the liberal opposition between the idealised figure of the rational, autonomous individual, and the devalued figure of the emotional, dependent person unable to think for themselves. "False memory" advocates described trustworthy and "true" memories as explicit, cognitive, persistent and recalled by individuals in isolation from other people. In contrast, untrustworthy memories involved any memory that departed from this standard, particularly where there was discontinuity in memory, where memory took implicit, embodied or affectively intensive forms, or where memory recollection was in some way "triggered" or facilitated by other events or people. These simple binaries of true/false, rational/emotional, continuous/discontinuous and independent/dependent were highly gendered and used to mischaracterise women seeking mental health care, in particular, as easily manipulated and incapable of judgement or independent thought (Gaarder, 2000).

These binaries were particularly salient in the 1990s during a period of neoliberal ascendency, in which individual self-sufficiency was valorised and dependency on others was pathologised. Sexual and civil libertarians accused the state and advocates for survivors of child abuse of exaggerating the problem, and the "false memory" narrative became the dominant child abuse "story" globally (Beckett, 1996; Kitzinger, 2004). Media bias was so widespread as to permanently distort the public record. For instance, lax regulation and oversight of the rapidly expanding daycare and childcare sectors had created new opportunities for sexual abusers to access children (Finkelhor & Williams, 1988). In some cases, centres were established for the explicit purpose of sexually exploiting children. In their zeal to advance an argument about false allegations and social hysteria, the forensic and other evidence for this chilling phenomena was pervasively misreported and suppressed (Cheit, 2014). Today, many believe that the 1980s and 1990s was a period of "daycare sex-abuse hysteria" (as one Wikipedia entry puts it), rather than a time where legal and policy failures exposed children in institutional settings to sexual violence and exploitation.

Mental health professionals, academics and advocates have attempted to right the record through strategic research and dissemination, as well as a critical questioning of "false memory" claims. Research into amnesia, dissociation and treatment for the effects of child abuse burgeoned during the 1990s (Brown et al., 1998), providing the basis for effective and evidence-based treatment of complex trauma. Researchers, clinicians and advocates documented flaws in the conduct of "false memory" research and its application to child abuse (e.g. Pope, 1996; Freyd, 1998). Media misrepresentations of cases of extreme abuse (such as organised or ritual abuse) were disputed by child protection and mental health professions working with profoundly traumatised clients (e.g. Sinason, 1994). It is telling, however, that this scholarship was almost wholly ignored by journalists and researchers aligned with the "false memory" position. There was no enthusiasm in the mass media for new research findings on trauma and abuse, or the debunking of previous journalistic claims about traumatic amnesia. To the contrary, "false memory" advocates were provided with extensive media and professional opportunities unrestrained by the accumulating evidence of exaggerations, over-generalisations and self-contradictions. Meanwhile, academics and professionals expressed their fear of speaking out against the "false memory" position, anticipating a public backlash (Kitzinger, 1998).

The disruption of the "false memory" narrative

Ultimately, what disrupted (although it did not displace) the false memory narrative was not science or data; it was another story. In 2002, the *Boston Globe* published a series of articles about clergy sexual abuse of children in the local Catholic diocese, triggering intense media coverage that eclipsed even the height of "false memory" reporting during the 1990s (Cheit, Shavit & Reiss-Davis, 2010). In direct refutation of "false memory" claims about social over-reaction to child sexual abuse, revelations of widespread clergy abuse were indicative of pervasive disinterest and inaction in relation to child sexual abuse, as well as high-level complicity amongst authorities. Subsequent scandals regarding the elite sexual deviance of UK entertainer Jimmy Savile, US coach Jerry Sandusky and other high-profile figures and celebrities (including those named in the current #MeToo movement) only underscored the degree of social toleration for child sexual offending.

Furthermore, in the aftermath of the global financial crisis (GFC), the liberal notion of the sovereign individual so central to "false memory" discourse has been challenged in significant ways. The GFC revealed the catastrophic narcissism of neoliberal individualism as well as the dense interconnectivity of economic and social relations, which operated to instantaneously transmit the consequences of the crisis around the world. In a post-GFC world, the ideal of the self-determining individual is now the terrain of significant social conflict. The "false memory" marriage of liberal individualism with scientism (in which the vocabulary and authority of science is appropriated for ideological or political purpose) was, in many respects, the forerunner to more explicitly reactionary contemporary movements (with varying labels, including overlapping bands of so-called "sceptics", "new atheists", "men's rights activists" and the "alt-right") in which a dogmatic positivism and individualism camouflages attempts to wind back the gains of the feminism, civil rights and other progressive social movements. Against this, a resurgent left asserts more socially embedded and accountable conceptualisations of individuality.

While its central tenets have been undermined, the "false memory" narrative remains an important journalistic touchstone. The tone of mass media coverage is generally more sympathetic to claims of child sexual victimisation than in the past, although journalists routinely warn against a return to the "satanic panics" and "witch hunts" of the 1980s and 1990s. This formulation seeks to retain the "false memory" narrative by "historicising" it, and re-imagining the 1980s and 1990s as a period of sexual neurosis that contemporary society has transcended and overcome, but must remember as a cautionary tale (Richardson, 2015). Arguably, this re-envisioning attempts to reconcile the contradictions between the popularity of the "false memory" narrative, and the accumulated evidence rendering that narrative untenable. As a result, the "false memory" story now co-exists uneasily alongside a renewed understanding of child sexual abuse as widespread, hidden and harmful.

Changing the narrative

It is important to ask why the "false memory" story was so influential for so long. Research offers some explanations. Kiztinger (2004) highlights the masculine culture of journalism, and suggests that, by the early 1990s, many (largely male) journalists and editors were already sceptical about abuse allegations and sympathetic towards accused men. Furthermore, she suggests that child abuse had become a "boring" and repetitive issue for journalists, who found the "false memory" story novel and appealing (Kitzinger, 1996). It is also useful to take political economy into consideration. The political climate of the 1980s and 1990s was, as previously explained, hostile to state services and intervention, and promoted a neoliberal ideology of personal autonomy that characterised claims of childhood trauma as an "excuse" for poor life outcomes. The figure of the adult woman "dependent" on a therapist was contrary to the ideal of the independent, autonomous individual that was implicitly championed in "false memory" science (Campbell, 2003) and in social and political discourse more broadly.

It is no accident that the "false memory" movement and narrative drew on these tendencies and sympathies. The brokers of this narrative, including people accused of abuse, and their academic and journalistic allies, were savvy in developing a story that "made sense" to the contemporary context. In doing so, they popularised a schema, or a way of making sense of the world, that did not supply new information about child abuse as much as it provided a new way of understanding child abuse altogether. In his book on the politics of storytelling, Monbiot (2017, p. 2) explains that:

> [w]hen we encounter a complex issue and try to understand it, what we look for is not consistent and reliable facts but a consistent and comprehensible story. When we ask ourselves whether something "makes sense", the "sense" we seek is not rationality, as scientists and philosophers perceive it, but narrative fidelity. Does what we are hearing reflect the way we expect humans and the world to behave? Does it hang together? Does it progress as stories should progress?

Child abuse was undoubtedly a complex issue about which little was known when it became a major media focus in the 1980s. The ubiquity of sexual abuse did not "fit" with community understandings of the benevolence of foundational social institutions, such as families, churches and schools. The undeniable predominance of male child sex offenders could be, and was, interpreted as an implicit critique of male sexuality, prompting defensiveness and claims of a feminist conspiracy amongst some men (Kitzinger, 2004). The bounds of journalistic and public credulity were stretched and ultimately exceeded by the controversial multiperpetrator, multi-victim abuse cases of the late 1980s and early 1990s (Salter, 2013, 2018). As these child abuse cases accumulated, they disrupted what Monbiot (2017) called "narrative fidelity" or "common sense" logic of the dominant story of child abuse as a "hidden epidemic". In its place, people accused of child abuse and their allies offered a story that seemed to progress much more sensibly, in which the severity of child abuse had been exaggerated, with many purported survivors suffering instead from "false memories". This story was embedded within, and consonant with, a broader set of beliefs and principles about individual autonomy and self-sufficiency that spoke to those collective anxieties evident during the period in which "false memory" claims were ascendant.

The scientific basis of the "false memory" narrative has always been poor. Fervent appeals to science and rationality in "false memory" discourse have not been matched with an equivalent commitment to scientific rigour (Pope, 1996; Freyd, 1998). A recent review has demonstrated the extent to which "false memory" research findings have been exaggerated, misapplied and over-generalised (Brewin & Andrews, 2017). It has been the narrative, rather than scientific, framework of "false memories" that explains both its enduring appeal and remarkable persistence in light of contradictory information. Monbiot (2017, p. 2) asserts that, once people believe a story that helps them make sense of the world, they will cling to this story even when shown that it is fictitious. He observes that "[a]ttempts to refute such stories tend only to reinforce them, as the disproof constitutes another reiteration of the narrative". His book includes numerous such examples: theories that American politicians orchestrated the disaster of 11 September, or that scientists are inventing climate change data for money, or that the private sector is more efficient and innovative than the public sector. Contrary evidence has not dislodged these narratives because they are part of a broader framework of meaning that has significance in people's lives. In the case of child abuse, the "false memory" narrative provided a façade of scientific justification for the appealing belief that child abuse was not as serious as victimised children and adults would suggest.

Of course, it is often necessary to specifically refute the points made to justify these exculpatory narratives; however, refutation is, alone, an insufficient response. Indeed, constant refutation transforms the disingenuous narrative into the grounds upon which debate takes place, and reinforces and disseminates (and strengthens) the narrative even more. Responding to the "false memory" narrative, then, walks a fine line between refutation and inadvertent reinforcement. Too much focus on contesting the claims of "false memory" advocates risks narrowing the discussion to "memory suggestibility" and the prevalence of false allegations, thus obscuring the broader social and political obstacles to the prevention, detection and treatment of child abuse. Rather than trying to counter stories with data, Monbiot (2017) emphasises the need for countervailing stories that give new coherence and meaning to the available information, and finds common cause amongst multiple actors and perspectives.

Trauma: a new story

It is interesting to note that, despite the prominence of the "false memory" narrative, the concept the concept of "trauma" has become more – not less – salient over the last 30 years. While there are legitimate critiques of the manner in which the concept of "trauma" pathologises suffering and grief, it is also the case that traumatic diagnoses such as post-traumatic stress disorder and dissociative identity disorder describe a shared array of human responses to degradation and dehumanisation (Good & Hinton, 2016; Ross, 2011). Trauma provides an accessible way of describing, and relating, to the universality of loss and betrayal and its impacts on human wellbeing, which has given the concept a great degree of resonance across the spectrum of personal and professional experience. The growing alliance and interweaving of neuroscience with trauma treatment and psychodynamic theory has fascinated the public, as evident in the runaway success of van der Kolk's (2015) bestselling book *The Body Keeps the Score*. Frameworks of "trauma-informed" practice have expanded beyond mental health services to a range of settings, including education, development and international aid, law enforcement and alcohol and drug services. Trauma has also become an important political concept. The vocabulary of intergenerational, collective and historical trauma has provided Indigenous and First Nations movements with ways of speaking about the ongoing impacts of colonisation, dispossession and genocide. In short, trauma is on the public agenda as never before.

The public understanding of trauma has developed to the point of offering a compelling, and ultimately, hopeful, counter-narrative to "false memory" disinformation. For a political narrative to be effective, Monbiot (2017, p. 13) says that it must be "simple and intelligible", "resonate with deep needs and desires", "explain the mess we are in and how to escape it", while being "firmly grounded in reality" and realistic solutions. All of these elements are evident in the contemporary field of trauma studies and treatment. As a concept, trauma speaks to the centrality of relationships to human flourishing, and what happens when that connectedness is interrupted, misused or broken. This deep need for mutual, nurturing relationships is made all the more acute within a social and economic environment that remains profoundly atomising and competitive. It might be said, with Alford (2016), that within a consumer culture that offers few resources to speak about or acknowledge suffering, "trauma" has become a crucially important placeholder for human vulnerability and loss. The very fact that "trauma" runs counter to the compulsory and exhausting optimism of a neoliberal focus on individual responsibility, competition and success may, at least partially, explain its increasing cultural footprint. "Trauma" reminds us of our fundamental dependence upon and openness towards others, and the subtle or overt wounds of misrecognition and maltreatment: whether due to misattunement or abuse between caregiver and child, or the dominations of misogyny, racism, class, imperialism and other axes of inequality.

Trauma treatment, research and discourse has affirmed the importance of emotionally rich, but not overwhelming or re-traumatising, relationships as the optimum condition for human flourishing, and for relational repair and restoration. This focus on intersubjectivity is, perhaps, the key "missing piece" of previous stories about child abuse. In the past, child abuse has been a problem without a solution, with distressing case after case accumulating in public awareness without apparent end. At least the "false memory" narrative offered a potential, if illusory and damaging, resolution to this intolerable situation, in the (re)suppression of victim complaints. However, there are now a number of promising pathways towards the prevention, detection and treatment of child sexual abuse amongst a host of other social problems. Congruent with the focus of trauma discourse on the strengthening of relationality, prevention efforts include parenting education and family support, child-safe institutions, community organising, well-resourced health, welfare and educational systems, and the promotion of economic and social equality, all of which reduce the risk of child sexual abuse amongst other forms of violence and maltreatment (Quadara et al., 2015). Trauma-informed responses to at-risk, victimised and/or perpetrating groups have a robust evidence base, and a crucial role to play in the amelioration of a range of social problems beyond child abuse. Major epidemiological studies such as the Adverse Childhood Experiences study have established the traumatic origins of social issues from crime and substance abuse to intergenerational disadvantage. In this sense, "trauma" does not only describe a problem but, increasingly, points in the direction of much-needed solutions.

Conclusion

The "Memory Wars" of the 1990s were a "trial by fire" for still-nascent attempts to develop evidence-based treatment of trauma and dissociative disorders. After a period of sustained media interest in child sexual abuse in the 1980s, "false memory" advocates were successful in reframing evidence of widespread sexual abuse as evidence of false allegations. In this process, the vocabulary of liberal individualism and scientific rationality was deployed in highly ideological ways against adults disclosing sexual abuse in childhood, and those mental health professionals who provided them with care. The narrative of "false memories" was based upon the public political impulses of the day, and provided journalists, academics and the public with a way of explaining the sudden increase in allegations of sexual abuse, particularly where those allegations challenged "common sense" understandings. A key advantage that "false memory" advocates enjoyed over their opponents was that research into child sexual abuse, and its traumatic effects, was in its infancy, whereas "false memory" advocates were championing a tradition of "scientific" disbelief in women's and children's allegations of sexual violence that dates back centuries. This tradition provided the "false memory" story with an appealing resolution: a return to familiar scepticism and silencing of sexual abuse complaints.

Advocates for child abuse survivors and trauma-informed treatment are often warned not to "go beyond the data" in asserting the credibility of abuse disclosures and therapeutic practice. While accurate information is a necessary part of the response to "false memory" disinformation, it is not sufficient on its own. The "false memory" story has persisted to the present day, albeit in a battered and somewhat revised form, because it has yet to be confronted by a counter-narrative of equivalent emotional and explanatory power. In this chapter, I've argued that psychological and political discourses of trauma provide the "raw material" for the construction of just such a narrative. In lay as well as professional understandings, trauma is being "storified" in a manner that appeals directly to our first-person experiences of relational connection and betrayal, affirming our deepest needs for attachment and human recognition. This narrative suggests that many individual and social problems originate in the neglect and abuse of human vulnerability, which must be repaired and protected. These claims are grounded in strong moral and empirical foundations, and they point to realistic solutions. Whereas the child abuse story has typically been one of despair, and the "false memory" narrative has been one of cynicism, the story of "trauma" is, increasingly, one of hope. Hopefulness emerges as a critically important principle for those seeking to inform the public not only about the problem of child abuse but also its solutions.

References

Alford, C. F. (2016). *Trauma, Culture, and PTSD*. London: Palgrave Macmillan.

Beckett, K. (1996). Culture and the Politics of Signification: The Case of Child Sexual Abuse. *Social Problems*, 43 (1), 57–76.

Brewin, C. R. & Andrews, B. (2017). Creating Memories for False Autobiographical Events In Childhood: A Systematic Review. *Applied Cognitive Psychology*, 31 (1), 2–23.

Brown, D., Scheflin, A. W. & Hammond, D. C. (1998). The Contours of the False Memory Debate. In D. Brown, A. W. Scheflin & D. C. Hammond (Eds.), *Memory, Trauma Treatment and the Law*. New York/London: W. W. Norton and Company, pp. 21–65.

Campbell, B. (2021) *Secrets and Silence: Child Sex Abuse from Cleveland to Savile and Beyond*. Bristol: Policy Press.

Campbell, S. (2003). *Relational Rremembering: Rethinking the Memory Wars*. Oxford: Rowman and Littlefield Publishers, Inc.

Cheit, R. (2014). *The Witch-Hunt Narrative: Politics, Psychology and the Sexual Abuse of Children*. Oxford: Oxford University Press.

Cheit, R. E., Shavit, Y. & Reiss-Davis, Z. (2010). Magazine Coverage of Child Sexual Abuse, 1992–2004. *Journal of Child Sexual Abuse*, 19 (1), 99–117.

Cooper, M. (2017). *Family Values: Between Neoliberalism and the New Social Conservatism*. New York: Zone Books.

Donaldson, L. J. & O'Brien, S. (1995). Press Coverage of the Cleveland Child Sexual Abuse Enquiry: A Source of Public Enlightenment? *Journal of Public Health*, 17 (1), 70–76.

Finkelhor, D. & Williams, L. M. (1988). *Nursery Crimes: Sexual Abuse in Day Care*. Newbury Park: Sage.

Finnane, M. & Smaal, Y. (2016). Some Questions of History: Prosecuting and Punishing Child Sexual Assault. In Y. Smaal, A. Kaladeflos & M. Finnane (Eds.), *The Sexual Abuse of Children: Recognition and Redress*. Clayton: Monash University Publishing, pp. 7–19.

Freyd, J. J. (1998). Science in the Memory Debate. *Ethics & Behavior*, 8 (2), 101–113.

Gaarder, E. (2000). Gender Politics: The Focus on Women in the Memory Debates. *Journal of Child Sexual Abuse*, 9 (1), 91–106.

Good, B. J. & Hinton, D. E. (2016). Introduction: Culture, Trauma and PTSD. In D. E. Hinton & B. J. Good (Eds.), *Culture and PTSD: Trauma in Global and Historical Perspective*. Pennsylvania: University of Pennsylvania Press, pp. 3–49.

Hechler, D. (1988). *The Battle and the Backlash: The Child Sexual Abuse War*. Toronto: Lexington Books.

Kitzinger, J. (1996). Media Representations of Sexual Abuse Risks. *Child Abuse Review*, 5 (5), 319–333.

Kitzinger, J. (1998). The Gender-Politics of News Production: Silenced Voices and False Memories. In C. G. Carter & S. Allan (Eds.), *News, Gender and Power*. London: Routledge, pp. 186–203.

Kitzinger, J. (2004). *Framing Abuse: Media Influence and Public Understanding of Sexual Violence against Children*. London/Ann Arbor: Pluto Press.

Monbiot, G. (2017). *Out of the Wreckage: A New Politics for an Age of Crisis*. London: Verso.

Olafson, E., Corwin, D. L. & Summit, R. C. (1993). Modern History of Child Sexual Abuse Awareness: Cycles of Discovery and Suppression. *Child Abuse & Neglect*, 17, 7–24.

Pope, K. S. (1996). Memory, abuse and science: Questioning claims about the false memory syndrome epidemic. *American Psychologist*, 51, 957–974.

Quadara, A., Nagy, V., Higgins, D. & Siegel, N. (2015). *Conceptualising the Prevention of Child Sexual Abuse: Final Report*. Sydney: Australian Institute of Family Studies. https://aifs.gov.au/sites/default/files/publication-documents/rr33.pdf

Richardson, K. (2015). Dissecting Disbelief: Possible Reasons for the Denial of the Existence of Ritual Abuse in the United Kingdom. *International Journal for Crime, Justice & Social Democracy*, 4 (2).

Ross, C. A. (2011). Possession Experiences in Dissociative Identity Disorder: A Preliminary Study. *Journal of Trauma & Dissociation*, 12 (4), 393–400.

Salter, M. (2013). *Organised Sexual Abuse*. London: Glasshouse/Routledge.

Salter, M. (2018) Organized Child Sexual Abuse in the Media. In H. Pontel (Ed.), *Oxford Research Encyclopedia of Criminology and Criminal Justice*. Oxford/ London: Oxford University Press.

Shengold, L. (2000). *Soul Murder Revisited: Thoughts about Therapy, Hate, Love, and Memory*. London: Yale University Press.

Sinason, V. (Ed.) (1994). *Treating Survivors of Satanist Abuse*. London: Routledge.

Van der Kolk, B. (2015). *The Body keeps the Score: Brain, Mind, and Body in the Healing of Trauma*. London: Penguin.

Chapter 14

"Do no harm"?

Khadija Rouf and Danny Taggart

Part I. Hearing and responding to victims and survivors

The themes of power, entrapment, shame and silence are central to child sexual abuse. No victim or survivor discloses into a neutral space, and there are many historical examples of how the testimony of survivors has been systematically discredited or ignored. This chapter examines how society reacts, and argues that there is a need for existing structures to change and become more trauma-informed. There is a need for ethical and just responding to ensure children are protected from abuse.

> To whom should I complain? Did I tell this,
> Who would believe me?
>> Isabella's monologue, *Measure for Measure*, Act 2, Scene 4,
>> William Shakespeare

We open with Isabella's plea, because her dilemma captures so much about power, abuse and entrapment. So often, survivors of abuse say that they thought they wouldn't be believed if they disclosed, or have had experiences of not being believed when they did tell.

We write from multiple, interconnected perspectives: as clinical psychologists engaged in working with survivors of abuse; as an academic studying the effects of trauma and working at the current UK Independent Inquiry into Child Sexual Abuse (IICSA) (Danny Taggart); and survivors of childhood sexual abuse ourselves. We have written and spoken about our experiences to widen the available narratives and to enrich and diversify the identities available to professionals and survivors (Rouf, 1989, 1990; Rouf & Rhodes, 2017; Taggart, 2016, 2017). Here, we draw on theory and evidence from applied psychology and social science to understand processes that drive some of the current debates about memory and abuse. We reflect on whether survivors have been treated ethically across time; how society reacts when disclosures happen; and how we can respond differently.

We argue that survivor voices have been marginalised and misrepresented and need to be placed at the heart of discussions. By listening to the phenomenological

DOI: 10.4324/9781003193159-15

experience of abuse survivors, we can reach a more socially just and ethically accountable position. Merely recognising the identity of survivors is only the first step; both restorative justice and redistribution of power are needed, to adequately protect children and to address the harm caused by abuse when it happens. In other words, we need to hear, believe and respond justly.

Introduction

Abuse is horrible. It is horrible to think about. Thinking about what a person is capable of doing to a child can be unbearable. Thinking about how power can be abused at the most intimate level and against the most vulnerable can be unbearable.

This can affect how society hears and responds to abuse disclosures. Societal responses are likely to be shaped by a number of influences, including public understandings of child abuse. Abuse compromises autonomy and dignity can impact on access to justice and can cause great harm (Rouf & Taggart, 2018). Whether society responds ethically and helpfully to address these injuries can depend on cultural consensus, which is open to shifts over time.

Historically, that cultural consensus has not been informed by victims, but rather powerful figures in science. The lived experiences of abuse survivors are often surrounded by secrecy, shame and silence. As a result, victims have been locked out of the narratives constructed about them, rather than with them. Persistent assumptions have been made about victims, about their credibility, motives, memories, their sexualities and capacities. Such assumptions can become normative, dominant and unquestionable. They can be invisible and influence the structures in which we live without our conscious awareness. They may make society feel "safe" by minimising abuse and placing it at a distance. And so, society remains in stasis, easily discarding the symbolism of individual reports of abuse. But such a stance can lead to secondary harm to victims via ignoring them, shaming, ostracising and silencing them. This does little to protect children.

In order to hear and respond ethically to victims and survivors, it is important to reflect on how ethics, ideology and history are intertwined, and are indelibly intertwined with power. The debate about the validity of survivor disclosures should be placed in a wider societal and historical narrative around child sexual abuse and collective responses to it. Societies are partly shaped by human psychology, and mirror those human biases. They are also shaped by time. As such, debates about memory need to take account of the social and political context in which science is conducted and communicated. This may require us to be shaken.

Historically, pendulum clocks were used to detect earthquakes: societal level shocks can cause crises in cultural consensus, leading the pendulum of public opinion to swing violently. Sometimes the societal understanding of abuse advances; sometimes, it swings backwards again. The distance of the swing reflects ambivalence about facing up to childhood sexual abuse. On the one hand, we want to protect our children and feel rage when they are harmed. On the other, disgust, fear and shame can shut down the ability to think, and can lead to denial. Neither of these positions keep children safe, as society fails to deal with the structural problems which facilitate abuse.

History suggests that we must study societal reactions to disclosures, in order to shock-proof structures and respond helpfully to victims and survivors. We can learn to anticipate, understand and work together to ensure that when structures are shaken, they do not collapse. To that end, survivors' accounts must reshape both architecture and process, to ensure ethical responses to disclosures. The creation of a Code of Ethics for victims and survivors of abuse could be a way of renovating the existing structure. It is an opportune time to end the silence, hostility and discrimination that victims of abuse often face.

The Foundations – history, ethics, power and psychology

> The most effective way to destroy people is to deny and obliterate their own understanding of their history.
>
> George Orwell (1949)

"Do no harm" is a central ethic of helping professionals. However, the history of applied ethics in the study and treatment of those with mental health problems is itself troubled. As clinicians, we understand the importance of establishing a coherent narrative between the past and present, in order to contextualise and understand distress. Similarly, it is helpful to contextualise responses to victims over time. Otherwise, powerful underlying assumptions remain invisible but dominant (Boyle, 2017 on ideological power).

Psychotherapy has been dominated by the trope of the "fantasist" victim, playing out an internal psychodrama of repressed desires (Freud, 1925). However, Freud initially believed disclosures of abuse made by his clients, and published work that supported this. The shock and backlash against him were immediate, and following ostracism, he retracted his findings and re-theorised, authoring the construct of "hysteria" (Masson, 1984). His professional power restored; he has become an iconic scientific figure.

Psychological theories then put bricks and mortar on these foundations. Victim disclosures were not heard, children were sexualised. The ideas had cultural capital, and were persistently repeated in many forms, in literature and media. In the 1970s and 1980s, there was active political lobbying by paedophiles for the abolition of the age of consent (Agerholm, 2016). In the 1990s, false memory discourse emerged and was quickly applied to child abuse, perhaps fitting part of an ingrained cultural narrative – to blame the victim by contesting the validity of their memories. It has also sought to discredit clinicians who work with survivors, and to conflate evidence and non-evidence-based therapies. These ideas gained a foothold in public attention.

It is feminist and survivor activism that has seriously challenged harmful narratives, offering a critique of power and placing survivor testimonies centrally. Another shift has occurred due to studying post-traumatic stress disorder (PTSD). Study into the experiences of those people who have suffered trauma has allowed an uncovering of its phenomenology. There is a growing body of evidence around the nature of trauma memories (Lancaster et al., 2016); single event trauma versus multiple traumas (Lancaster et al., 2016); the impacts of trauma in children (Mannarino et al., 2012) and evidence-based treatments (e.g. Ehlers et al., 2003). These findings expand understandings of memory and suggest that the extrapolation of "laboratory to real life" research findings regarding false memories may have been overstated (Brewin & Andrews, 2016).

Returning to ethics, we must consider whether history and science has treated victims fairly. Ethical principles concerning autonomy, client best interests, justice and avoidance of harm (Beauchamp & Childress, 2001) need renewal for work with survivors, particularly in a healthcare context that increasingly views patients as consumers engaging in a transaction.

Abuse and trauma responses are societal problems, not only individual, psychological or medical ones. This means societal level responsibility for trauma. The ethics of a "politics of recognition" alone might not go far enough (Fraser, 2003) in merely destigmatising the "spoiled" identity of the abuse survivor. Restorative practices for the survivor, redistribution of resources and wider systemic change are needed. Clinicians and researchers need to consider all levels of healing: psychological, physical, interpersonal, social and material. Scientific disputes about memory, while important, can distract from these wider issues of personal and political justice and mask society's responsibilities to victims.

History tells us that ethics, power and psychology are intertwined. Human narratives have shaped them – they are of their time; they are subject to social pressures and understandings; they are subject to prejudices, heuristics and flaws, e.g. Kahneman et al (1982). Clinicians need to reflect constantly on whether they are congruent with the stance, "Do no harm". A central part of this must be hearing and responding to survivors, including those who are from under-served or mis-served communities. This requires a different way of seeing, one which requires scrutiny of contexts.

Letting light into darkened rooms

> When I give food to the poor, they call me a saint. When I ask why the poor have no food, they call me a communist.
>
> Hélder Câmara, *Essential Writings* (see McDonagh, 2009)

Clinicians are trained to listen. It is important to be aware of factors that can affect our ability to listen to victims. Embedded assumptions and stereotypes can affect us without our awareness and will merely reflect those that pre-exist in and permeate society (Pearce & Cronen, 1980). Such assumptions may affect whether we engage in routine enquiry about abuse (Read, Hammersley & Rudegeair et al.,

2007), and they can impact on how we hear disclosures. Thus, disclosures may fit into pre-existing schema, a template of victimhood that misses the idiosyncrasies of individual stories.

It is our view that societal reactions to abuse reveal hidden schema, mythologies that can only serve to perpetuate abuse. These assumptions include, "Abuse is distal to us, and impossible in cherished institutions"; "It doesn't happen in nice, white, middle-class homes"; "It's perpetrated by a few weird individuals, rather than a problem with toxic masculinity"; "Those who disclose are 'mad' or 'seeking attention'". Research shows the heightened vulnerabilities of children from backgrounds with intersecting "minority" identities; the perceptions about "who victims are" can render children invisible if they have disabilities, are from BAME, LGBTQ backgrounds or are male (Fox, 2016). These hierarchies of vulnerability mean that there are groups of people in society who are persistently under-served, mis-served and marginalised, often on a daily basis. Why should these victims and survivors trust a society which repeatedly breaks its social contract with them?

We must be conscious of the pressures exacted on survivors. Abuse is still a highly taboo subject; even though mental health problems are being destigmatised and normalised, the underlying injuries are not (Taggart & Speed, 2019). Survivors can find it highly shaming and frightening to disclose. There are a multitude of common themes regarding why people cannot talk about abuse (e.g. Peake & Fletcher, 1997), and also highly personal and idiosyncratic reasons. Not enough attention is paid to the reasons why people cannot tell or are unable to tell for a long period of time. Where there has been silence, the meaning of this silence has often been misrepresented – as indicative of "lies", "fantasy", "false memory" – and is harmful. As clinicians, these embedded tropes may affect our practice, our ability to hear and believe.

The systems in which we practice may also reflect the pressures not to disrupt societal structures. This includes the research which informs practitioners: what is up for scientific study is not a neutral decision; how those scientific findings are interpreted may not be a neutral endeavour. While it may be important for clinicians to take up a position of strategic neutrality in working with suspected abuse, it will come at a cost for survivors; not being believed will be familiar to many and they may struggle with the consequences of institutional doubt. If organisations are not trauma-informed, then this can lead to structural oppression of victims (Sweeney et al., 2016; Sweeney & Taggart, 2018). Power imbalances may be coded into the wording of appointment letters, the layout of waiting rooms, the availability (or not) of services which give time and space for people to express their stories. Again, we reflect on "who owns the story?" of what happened to a victim. In their attempts to seek help, victims may have to tell their story many times over. They may be ignored, misheard, partially heard and interpreted in ways that are not faithful to their experiences. Survivors risk being mis-labelled as "mad or bad" and denied access to suitable forms of help and justice. All these reasons can mean it is simply not safe enough for people to tell.

How can we open the curtains in darkened spaces to spotlight injustice? Can we ask questions that take us beyond the familiar confines of the therapy room? Such questions include:

- "Why don't we see the abuse of women and children as a form of hate crime?"
- "How does societal power render some groups particularly vulnerable to abuse?"
- "How do we prevent the social exclusion, out-grouping and othering of victims?"

These questions can be answered more clearly if we listen to what survivors have to say.

What survivors can teach us – there are stories in the walls

There is no greater agony than bearing an untold story inside you.

Maya Angelou (1984)

Researchers studying trauma are building a body of work about its impact. Abuse is harmful: the link between childhood sexual abuse and psychiatric disorder is strongly causal, particularly for psychosis (Bentall et al., 2012). Adverse childhood experiences (ACEs) have multifactorial negative impacts on health and wellbeing (Felitti & Anda, 2009). Work with trauma survivors is revealing that symptoms of traumatic injury can include hyperarousal; disruptions to the usual processes of remembering and forgetting (intrusive memories, flashbacks, nightmares, dissociation); heightened levels of avoidance; shattered assumptions about the self, world and others; and an association with a range of diagnoses, such as depression (Chapman et al., 2004) and self-destructive behaviours, such as suicidality (Dube et al., 2001). However, even this body of work may miss what it is like to live through interpersonal violation and what Freyd (1994) has called Betrayal Trauma; perpetrators exert power and pressure not to tell, and impose distorted interpretations of events upon their victims.

Trauma impacts on when people tell – it can take years to disclose and seek help, and also how people tell – they "often tell their stories in a highly emotional, contradictory, and fragmented manner" (Herman, 2015, p. 1). Traumatic injuries weave into subjective experience, moulding perceptions of our identities, our bodies, other people and the world in myriad microscopic and structural ways. The effort to bring this to awareness, never mind words, is enormous. Survivor narratives offer an all-encompassing sense of what it is to be "in" trauma in a way that clinical descriptors of "trauma" cannot. The phenomenology of trauma must, therefore, be led by survivor owned stories, which are treated with dignity.

The *secondary injury* caused when society responds pathologically towards victims and survivors is also a neglected part of the story. Victims are scrutinised, their words are called into question. But there are gaps in scientific enquiry. For instance, there appears little scrutiny of the memory of alleged perpetrators. Also, little attention is focused on how family, community or societal responses can either heal trauma or amplify its impact.

We have already mentioned the harms caused by stereotyping and heuristics. Some victims may endure identity based prejudice, such as racism or sexism, because of who they are. But victims may also face discrimination at an embodied level because of what happened to them. They may endure rejection, disbelief or be subject to fatalistic "terminal diagnosis" narratives about recovery, which rob them of possibilities for post-traumatic growth or a positive future life. If victims are labelled, then we must consider the wider context and who is doing this labelling, and why.

Societal shock reactions – responding to victims by bolting the doors?

> The ordinary response to atrocities is to banish them from consciousness.
>
> Herman (2015, p. 1)

Societal systems provide institutional authority and resources to behave as they do (Zimbardo 2007; Smail, 2005); our responses are shaped by those systems at every layer of interaction, consciously and unconsciously (Pearce & Cronen, 1980). So, it is crucial we examine societal level responses to abuse. Again, history suggests that society's relationship with the existence of interpersonal violence is an uneasy one; there are silences and denials of abuse, tropes that victim blame, undermine victim testimony and attack people who support victims either personally or professionally. Erasure and collective forgetting are ordinary responses; this is why there are movements to ensure collective remembering in the wake of mass violence, such as the Holocaust and the Rwandan Genocide. If we do not remember, learn, reconcile and heal, then we may be destined to repeat.

Historically, cultural consensus has not been victim informed. Perhaps, victim disclosures create a cognitive dissonance that threatens our sense of an orderly, safe world. As a consequence, survivors are pushed to the margins, pressured not to speak out and sanctioned if they do. This can include social, cultural and familial rejection, financial hardships, being called a "liar", being called "mad", being driven "mad"; promoting fatalistic attitudes about their capacities to function in society. These forms of social exclusion can be understood as out-grouping (Tajfel & Turner, 1979, 1986). This exposes victims to secondary injuries.

When societal shock reactions occur, such as after the exposure of large-scale abuse, our sense of time and place can be thrown out of equilibrium. The interplay of changes can throw the pendulum into violent swing and dysregulation. The patterns contain repeated themes: fear and disbelief; denial and victim-blaming; "recognition" of abuse and a shift towards outrage; trial by media; demonisation and "othering"/out-grouping of suspected perpetrators; "reactivity" involving public concern and lengthy inquiry; "resolution" including "learning the lessons" (with individual-level account-ability and scapegoating) but often without structural change; "collective forgetting". Repeat.

These reactions occur during periods of high stress, and as such, decisions are more likely to depend on stereotypes or heuristics (Taylor, 2004). If it occurs "far away", geographically or socially, we can safely distance our world from it. If abuse is proximal, people can be fearful and disoriented, as though they have lost their sense of normality. Abuse being brought to light, close to home, shakes the foundations of family, community and society. This can lead to a conflation of healthy and abusive behaviour, which serves to fog and distract from the real issues of addressing harm, e.g. people expressing fears about cuddling children, as if they cannot recognise the parameters of abusive behaviour. Discourse falls into heated binaries, often resorting to highly emotive language. Positions shift back and forth, an example being the police's stance towards hearing and believing victims of abuse before doubting again (Laville, 2016).

It's important to understand the patterns, in order to anticipate them, to prevent potentially catastrophic responses towards victims and to take for-ward actions to protect children and vulnerable adults. Lessons learned should not lead to repeated themes. As clinicians, we need to understand the pendulum swing without becoming disoriented.

Shame plays a central role in the process: it is a profoundly physical response, leading to avoidance, denial, reflective paralysis, inability to articulate experience and the shutting down of discussion (Gilbert, 2010). Shame can be internal, external or reflected (Gilbert, 1998; Gilbert et al., 2004). Survivors are silenced by explicit or implicit societal messages that blame them for being abused, or for making their injuries visible. This is connected to social withdrawal and ostra-cism. Shame is associated with a number of psychiatric problems (Thibodeau, Kim & Jorgensen, 2011). With limited choices and power, victims are forced to manage distress in unhealthy ways, and suffer further marginalisation.

At a societal level, collective shame may be avoided by projecting these feel-ings into perpetrators, but also professionals tasked with preventing abuse. Clin-icians may be scapegoated for "implanting" abuse memories and causing "moral panic". Society may also reject survivors – a form of societal "double-neglect" involving failure to respond to abuse in the first place, followed by a rejection if the survivor breaches the social contract; homelessness, substance dependence, "madness", struggling to work or parent, are all circumstances that are more likely following abuse. They also lead to community ostracism and the masking of survivor status behind psychiatric or antisocial diagnosis (typically as "per-sonality disorder").

This is where stereotyping can become hardwired into structures such as psy-chiatry; by locating the problem in the individual's personality, society does not take responsibility for changing structures in order to prevent harm. Stereotypes become hardwired into scientific endeavour, with avoidance of examining areas that are "too controversial" or "political". They become hardwired into legal processes, leading to low levels of legal justice for victims, and courtroom practices which subject victims to intolerable levels of hostile cross-examination, as in the case of Frances Andrade (Walker, 2013) and more recently in victims of sexual exploitation in Newcastle (Spicer, 2018).

As with shame, many of the micro-processes associated with one person's experience of abuse and its aftermath are mirrored at a societal level. Again, society has created narratives about survivors which are stereotypical, myth-based and heuristic. These are persistent, prevent disclosure and emerge at times of shock. Victims may be caught in binaries of "good" and "bad", their stories seen as either "credible" or "manipulative"; they may be viewed as psychologically doomed. Even the developing "survivor" narrative is simplistic, couched in individual "triumph over adversity"; this can inadvertently blame those who only partially survive, or do not survive at all. Simplified heuristics prevent adequate helping responses and lead to unethical responding.

Whilst harmful social responses exist, unhealthy societal responses are not inevitable. There is reason for optimism that society can become more understanding, empathic and adopt healthier, healing responses towards survivors. If systems become shock-proofed, then the swings that occur at the societal level can be less violent and disruptive.

Responding to shocks – the building should shake, not fall down

> Turning and turning in the widening gyre; the falcon cannot hear the falconer; things fall apart, the centre cannot hold; mere anarchy is loosed upon the world.
>
> W. B. Yeats (2000)

Shock-proofing systems means recognising the myriad ways that abuse can occur, taking structural action to prevent it and facilitating effective interventions to ameliorate it. Reason (1998, 2000) has written extensively on his "Swiss cheese" model of risk and safety in industrial settings. Catastrophic events can occur when there is failure at each level, perhaps starting with a seemingly small error, the consequences of which travel through different layers of an organisation, like the holes in Swiss cheese. The seemingly small, unchecked errors can gather momentum and have catastrophic consequences. This is a particular risk in "command and control" cultures, where there are big differentials in power. Human factors can have profound impacts; Munro's (1996, 1999) analysis of serious case reviews in child protection identifies errors, and highlights that clinician thinking biases, such as groupthink and over-optimism, can lead to catastrophic outcomes for children.

Zimbardo (2007) highlights how groups exert subtle pressures through their implied norms. He highlights factors, which can allow abuse to occur, include a lack of personal responsibility or anonymity; a habit of obedience/compliance/conformity to authority; high need for group approval and fear of ostracism;

passivity; command and control cultures without appropriate checks and balances; dehumanisation and small shifts which make abuses gradually seem "normal".

It is possible to make systems safer. Reason outlines that safe cultures have five features – they are informed; they facilitate safe reporting (without fear of blame); they learn from positive and negative feedback; they are just; and they are flexible. Safe cultures depend on trust, a non-blaming attitude to unintended mistakes, shared values and a sense of individual responsibility. Zimbardo (2007) outlines ways to reduce abuse, and clear values and ethics are key. Other features are being mindful of heuristics, having space to reflect, promoting altruism, and a just and diverse culture.

These myriad risk and protective factors can be reduced to platitudes and axioms, but can also be structured to shock-proof systems tasked with preventing and responding to abuse. This could form a type of critical incident planning. As clinicians, we have suggestions as to how these principles can be applied. As survivors, we have demands for a more victim-focused ethics.

Renovating the architecture – sometimes, it is time for structures to change

> Not everything that is faced can be changed. But nothing can be changed until it is faced ... Most of us are about as eager to change as we were to be born, and go through our changes in a similar state of shock.
>
> Baldwin (2011)

To reiterate, societal level shocks can shake the cultural consensus, leading the pendulum of public opinion to swing violently. Sometimes, efforts to "solve" those shocks are reactive, febrile, leading only to superficial change. We fail to acknowledge that it may be the very house we inhabit, our home, our way of living, which is a source of harm.

To acknowledge this is painful. It takes courage to do so. We still need shelter, and we need to belong. The house shakes, and this can spark fear that it will fall down entirely. But this shaking is also an opportunity for change – not only to imagine but to *realise* moving to a new equilibrium. Change may signal threat, but it is also a chance to achieve something deeper, with different underpinnings and new architecture; knocking out old walls, putting in new doors, changing the shape of the space within and letting in light.

1   *Work to illuminate the phenomenology of victimhood*

Clinicians are trained to listen, to respond empathically, to work collaboratively. We listen to stories, and we help people to reformulate and retell those stories. If someone has been abused and has internalised toxic messages which pervade daily life and blight their psychological landscape, then we work together to see new perspectives. This is a nuanced process. It involves hearing. The retelling of the narrative is a shared endeavour, which must be carefully done, which must be respectful of power and not impose yet another reality upon already harmful tropes.

We have a responsibility to reflect on how cultural messages may affect our work, and to correct harmful stereotypes about survivors. We can ensure we engage in routine enquiry about abuse (Read, Hammersley & Rudegeair, 2007), that we hear disclosures of non-recent abuse and take them seriously, and consider if there are potential current risks to children. Responding to disclosures can have therapeutic value if done sensitively and compassionately (British Psychological Society, 2016; Waites & Rouf, 2014). We can encourage the systems we work within to meaningfully hear the voices of victims and survivors. By adopting an approach that includes the potential for post-traumatic growth, we can assist someone on a path towards hope, healing and thriving.

2   A trauma-informed Code of Ethics

To our knowledge, there is no trans-disciplinary Code of Ethics that exists to address the issues faced by victims and survivors of abuse. We consider the creation of a Code to be necessary and that it could be helpful if adopted by institutions. This would not be designed to replace existing codes but to address the particular concerns faced by survivors. Feminist ethics outlines helpful key principles regarding therapist knowledge and accountability (competence), addressing cultural diversities and oppressions and working for egalitarian therapist–client relationships (Enns, 1996). Such a Code could work in line with professional codes and position statements (e.g. HCPC, 2016; BPS, 2014), Human Rights legislation, and the Convention of the Rights of the Child (United Nations, 1989). We envision that it would be co-produced with survivors, and shared with any survivor coming forward for help, so that they could be confident about their rights and expected ethical standards from services. (Please see Part 2 for a proposed outline.)

3   Shine light on power and structure

Structures can contain features that are weighted against certain groups. Ahmed (2017) articulates how this can operate from individuals to systems,

> An individual man who violates you is given permission: that is structure. His violence is justified as natural and inevitable: that is structure. A girl is made responsible for his violence: that is structure. A policeman who turns away because it is a domestic call: that is structure. A judge who talks about what she was wearing: that is structure. A structure is an arrangement, an order, a building, an assembly.
>
> (p. 30)

We must pay close attention to structural inequalities as these impact on survivor experiences – the victims who are invisible because they are boys; the young gay person who is frightened to disclose in case they suffer homophobic attack; the Asian woman who is rendered invisible, because staff do not understand the barriers she faces in disclosing; the disabled person who is not heard, because the mental health team building does not have adequate disabled access. These are scenarios involving structural failures to reach out to victims. Who is absent? Who is missing or marginalised from the social space?

The structure needs to change, the bricks and mortar, the policies, the mindsets. Clinicians can adapt practices so that victims are not just expected to contort themselves to "fit" into available narratives.

One story cannot capture many voices; there must be room for pluralism. There are fellow survivors who remain marginalised and do not have adequate access to the means to be heard. This needs to change. Considering intersectionality and the layers of adversities people endure is necessary to explore and map out the range of experiences of abuse and their aftermath, not only quantitatively but also utilising subjective, phenomenological methodologies. We, therefore, move away from a simplified heuristic of a "victim" and embrace a broader range of narratives, which include multiple forms of survival and resistance.

4 Work to shock-proof the environment

It is imperative that society develops architecture to withstand shocks and respond adequately to prevent and respond to abuse and its aftermath (almost as a form of critical incident planning). We need to acknowledge child abuse as a public health issue (Fellitti & Anda, 2009; Children's Commissioner, 2015) and as an issue of social justice.

Preparedness involves developing a non-blaming culture; where high value is placed on reflection, knowledge and learning; where ethics and justice underpin everything; and that is flexible and responsive. Such structures flatten out hierarchical power, recognising the potential harm of command and control cultures (Reason, 2000). The system needs to acknowledge that abuse happens and it happens on a significant scale. It needs to be able to hear anything about anyone, and to respond healthily to what it hears. Systems designed to help survivors should be co-produced with them (meaning not one or two survivors at the table, but collectives or representatives of collectives). It also means noticing which chairs at the table are empty, who never even gets as far as a place at the table. Under-served and mis-served communities need to have their voices heard, but gaining their trust to do so, requires humility, recognition of harm and building restorative relationships.

Shock-proofing requires rehearsing scenarios across the organisation, which can help to "drill" staff on how to respond. Examples of culture change are emerging, such as strategic plans to ensure health staff are trauma-informed, and that there are a range of skills for working with survivors (NHS Scotland, 2017).

Shock-proofing oneself is also essential; one may personally encounter resistance and hostility by association with what society may actively wish to forget. This means developing resilience to micro-aggressions, dealing with organisational resistance to change, or macro-aggressions such as attempts to cause reputational damage.

Be persistent, be prepared for the long haul, and ensure that social connection and work-life balance are part of self-care. It is important not to work in isolation, and keep an eye on the process – the swings are predictable. Changing structures is effortful. Wherever possible, celebrate successes.

5 Applied ethics in action – working to change foundations and structures

Acknowledging the scale of abuse invites a serious consideration of where to place professional energy. There is a tendency for therapy to happen in a social vacuum (Smail, 2005). Some clinicians will prefer to work on with individual clients or groups. Some may consider adopting approaches that talk about power and trauma as alternative narratives for survivors (Power Threat Meaning; Johnstone & Boyle, 2018). And some may widen their roles, and venture out of the therapy room and consider social action-based interventions.

Social action is designed to move from individual suffering to social change. One example, Holland's work with Bangladeshi women in London (Holland, 1992) began with a conventional individual therapy, but moved into group work, and then into a political activism. Abuse and consequential trauma can be framed as a psychological problem for individual sufferers and their families, a social problem that connects disparate individuals through a shared experience of victimisation, and also a political problem in the way that power operates to marginalise survivors while protecting abusers.

The way out of harm into healing involves the development of more nuanced narratives of abuse, survival and resistance. Survivors can develop forms of healing through collective action that reaches beyond clinical settings. Examples include indigenous women's practice of "parrhesia" involving "external attachment to larger social-political meanings rather than self-disclosure as narrative leading to diagnosis in a psychological truth" (Million, 2013, p. 89). Sociotherapy in Rwanda (Jansen et al., 2015) and survivor-led organisations such as the National Association for People Abused in Childhood (NAPAC), Survivors Trust and Rape Crisis England & Wales show how collective survivor voices might eschew typical "therapeutic" heuristics and enable different forms of healing. There are also partnerships between third sector organisations lobbying for systemic improvements, e.g. Manchester Survivors, Survivors UK, Mankind UK and Safeline, which are working together to improve responses to male survivors.

A key development in the UK context is the undertaking of inquiries into abuse across the Four Nations; England, Northern Ireland, Scotland and

Wales. At one time, this scale of inquiry would have been unimaginable, and it is notable that there are other countries undertaking their own investigations into the mass abuses of children.

The Independent Inquiry into Child Sexual Abuse started in 2015 and, at the time of writing, is ongoing. This inquiry was a response to a number of scandals, including the revelations about Jimmy Savile and the child sexual exploitation cases in Rotherham. In both of these cases, institutional failings were identified in not protecting children and in not taking seriously the testimony of victims. The inquiry was established on the basis of societal shocks, leading to a pendulum swing towards outrage and recrimination. But it offers the possibility of something different, and deeper, emerging.

Following the conclusion of a similar investigation into child sexual abuse and institutional failings in Australia, The Royal Commission, the sociologist Katie Wright (2018) proposes inquiries can be forms of Transitional Justice, whereby survivors can be listened to, and their claims believed. This can lead the discourse of trauma to be a recognised medium to agitate for wider social and political change. From this vantage point then the IICSA can offer survivors, public servants who work with them and wider society an opportunity to participate in a democratically informed process that contributes to "broader understandings of justice as both deeply personal and intrinsically social" (Wright, 2018, p. 190). This moves the type of justice available to survivors beyond the testimonial and therapeutic justice sanctioned by listening and believing accounts of child sexual abuse, and creates a discourse whereby wider forms of economic and social justice can emerge.

One example is the ongoing reform of the UK welfare system, whereby people unable to work as a result of disability are increasingly being punished by a harsh and confusing system of sanctioning, designed to reinstall them into a precarious labour market. This process of sanctioning has been found to have life-threatening consequences for many (Mehta et al., 2017) and carries significant risks of re-traumatisation and material deprivation. Given the findings of the ACEs research discussed at the beginning of this chapter, many people caught up in the welfare system will have suffered significant trauma in childhood, leading to ill health and disability, rendering them unable to "compete" in an insecure labour market. Remembering the institutional and societal failings that are the backdrop of abuse and its injurious aftermath for victims, how can we justify the secondary harm of punishing people and denying them access to basic resources to live?

Societal responsibility for providing justice and reparation to child sexual abuse survivors extends far beyond offering therapeutic amelioration and recognition of a stigmatised identity. It requires a radical reappraisal about how we respond to adversity and a rebalancing of resources to recognise (i.e. to hear, see, understand and respond to) the social and economic impact abuse has across the lifespan. It involves thoughtful, dynamic and expanded forms of justice, which again, involve hearing; access to help; being treated like a fellow human being (McGlynn & Westmarland, 2019).

Social responsibility must then lead to deep and meaningful social action. This opens up opportunities to work with survivor organisations, lobby decision makers, and campaign for improvements. There are victim informed shifts, such as the Victim Directive (European Parliament, 2012) and Istanbul Convention (Council of Europe, 2011), which the UK has yet to ratify but is being lobbied to do so. There have been advances in the treatment of vulnerable witnesses in court, but far more is needed if we are to see improvements in social and legal justice for victims. The 2030 Agenda for Sustainable Development Goals (United Nations, 2015) includes the aim of eradicating violence against women and girls (VAWG) across the planet. There is hope for transformational change, and we can all play our part in positively shifting the cultural consensus.

Conclusion

We write at a time when the collective disclosures of survivors are shifting societal perceptions about the scale of abuse. The landscape in the UK has shifted dramatically in light of high-profile cases, such as the Savile inquiry. All stories spotlight abuse perpetrated by powerful and trusted figures, whose access to institutional power gave them chances to abuse multiple victims for years. Collective disclosures of abuse are also being accompanied by a renewal of survivor-led activism, and social movements, like #MeToo, are sparking energy for change at a public health level (O'Neill et al., 2018).

Survivor accounts, combined with scientific advances in the understanding of trauma, are creating enriched understandings of how abuse can injure the usual process of memory and psychological functioning. Time is yielding an opportunity to reshape public understandings of trauma and its aftermath. This could lead to the correcting of harmful narratives which have led to unethical treatment of survivors, through denial, victim-blaming, or "othering". Systems designed to help should be careful not to compound the pressures on survivors. There is an opportunity to reshape structure to prevent societal responses which may amplify harm.

Chronological time, ideology, history and ethics are all part of this story. The clock ticks, shocks occur, the pendulum swings in the aftermath. If we learn to understand how the pendulum swings at a societal level, we can shock-proof structures and respond in ways that are socially just and ethical. We must strive to fight sensationalism and the temporary nature of stories that capture media attention, but ultimately serve only to protect power and preserve vulnerability.

Whilst the pendulum swings wildly, we must methodically and persistently get on with hearing and helping children and adults who have suffered abuse. They must be allowed to own their narratives, and we must do no harm. Those survivor-led narratives must be used to renew structure, process and establish a new equilibrium, a trauma-informed cultural consensus. There is a moment now.

In the words of current campaigners, *Time's up.*

References

Ahmed, S. (2017). *Living a Feminist Life*. Durham: Duke University Press.

Agerholm, H. (Friday 1 July2016). Founding Member of Paedophile Lobbying Group That Wanted to Lower Age of Consent Jailed for 24 years. *The Independent*.

Angelou, M. (1984). *I Know Why the Caged Bird Sings*. London: Virago.

Baldwin, J. (2011). *The Cross of Redemption: Uncollected Writings*. Randall Kenan (Ed.). New York: Vintage International Original.

Beauchamp, T. L. & Childress, J. F. (2001). *Principles of Biomedical Ethics*. Oxford: Oxford University Press.

Bentall, R. P.*et al.* (2012). "Do Specific Early-Life Adversities Lead to Specific Symptoms of Psychosis? A Study from the 2007 The Adult Psychiatric Morbidity Survey". *Schizophrenia Bulletin*, 38 (4), 734–740.

Boyle, M. (2017). *Power and Threat*. Paper presented as part of symposium "The Power/Threat/Meaning Framework", DCP Annual Conference, Liverpool.

Brewin, C. R. & Andrews, B. (2016). Creating Memories for False Autobiographical Events in Childhood: A Systematic Review. *Applied Cognitive Psychology*. doi:10.1002/acp.3220

British Psychological Society (BPS). (2016). *Guidance on the Management of Disclosures of Non-Recent (Historic) Child Sexual Abuse*. Leicester: BPS.

British Psychological Society. (2014). *Safeguarding and Promoting the Welfare of Children. Position Paper*. Leicester: BPS.

Chapman, D. P., Whitfield, C. L., Felitti, V. J., Dubea, S. R., Edwards, V. J. & Anda, R. F. (2004). Adverse childhood experiences and the risk of depressive disorders in adulthood. *Journal of Affective Disorders*, 82, 217–225.

Children's Commissioner. (2015). *Protecting Children from Harm: A Critical Assessment of Child Sexual Abuse in the Family Network in England and Priorities for Action*. London: Children's Commissioner for England.

Council of Europe. (2011). Council of Europe Convention on preventing and combating violence against women and domestic violence. Istanbul Convention. *Council of Europe Treaty Series*, 210, Istanbul, 11.V.2011.

Dube, S. R., Anda, R. F., Felitti, V. J., Chapman, D.P., Williamson, D. F. & Giles, W. H. (2001). Childhood Abuse, Household Dysfunction, and the Risk of Attempted Suicide Throughout the Life Span: Findings from the Adverse Childhood Experiences Study. *JAMA*, 26; 286 (24), 3089–3096.

Ehlers, A., Clark, D. M., Hackmann, A., Mcmanus, F., Fennell, M., Herbert, C. & Mayou, R. (2003). A Randomized Controlled Trial of Cognitive Therapy, a Self-Help Booklet, and Repeated Assessments as Early Interventions for Post-Traumatic Stress Disorder. *Archives of General Psychiatry*, 60, 1024–1032.

Enns, C. Z. (1996). The Feminist Therapy Institute Code of Ethics: Implications for Working with Survivors of Child Sexual Abuse. *Women and Therapy*, 19 (1), 79–92.

European Parliament. (2012). The Victims' Rights Directive 2012/29/EU. https://eur-lex.europa.eu/legal-content/EN/TXT/?uri=CELEX:32012L0029.

Felitti, V. J. & Anda, R. F. (2009). The relationship of adverse childhood experiences to adult health, well-being, social function, and healthcare. In: R. Lanius & E. Vermetten (Eds.), *The Hidden Epidemic: The Impact of Early Life Trauma on Health and Disease*. Cambridge: Cambridge University Press.

Fox, C. (2016). *"It's not on the Radar": The Hidden Diversity of Children and Young People at Risk of Sexual Exploitation in England*. London: Barnados.

Fraser, N. (2003). Social Justice in the Age of Identity Politics: Redistribution, Recognition, and Participation. In N. Fraser & A. Honneth (Eds.), *Redistribution or Recognition? A Political-Philosophical Exchange*. London: Verso, pp. 7–110.

Freud, S. (1925). An Autobiographical Study. In *Standard Edition*. London: Hogarth Press.

Freyd, J. J. (1994). Betrayal Trauma: Traumatic Amnesia as an Adaptive Response to Childhood Abuse. *Ethics and Behaviour*, 4 (4), 307–329.

Gilbert, P. (1998). What is shame? Some core issues and controversies. In P. Gilbert & B. Andrews (Eds.), *Shame: Interpersonal Behavior, Psychopathology and Culture*. New York: Oxford University Press, pp. 3–38.

Gilbert, P., Gilbert, J. & Sanghera, J. (2004). A Focus Group Exploration of the Importance Of Izzat, Shame, Subordination and Entrapment on Mental Health Service Use in South Asian Women Living in Derby. *Mental Health, Religion & Culture*, 7 (2), 109–130. doi:10.1080/13674670310001602418

Gilbert, P. (2010). An Introduction to Compassion Focused Therapy in Cognitive Behavior Therapy. *International Journal of Cognitive Therapy*, 3 (2), 97–112. doi:10.1521/ijct.2010.3.2.97

Herman, J. (2015). *Trauma and Recovery*. New York: Basic Books.

Holland, S. (1992). From Social Abuse to Social Action: A Neighbourhood Psychotherapy and Social Action Project for Women. In J. Ussher & P. Nicholson (Eds.), *Gender Issues in Clinical Psychology*. London: Routledge.

HCPC. (2016). *Standards of Conduct, Performance and Ethics*. London: Health and Care Professions Council.

Jansen, S., White, R., Hogwood, J., Jansen, A., Gishoma, D., Mukamana, D. & Richters, A. (2015). The "Treatment Gap" in Global Mental Health Reconsidered: Sociotherapy for Collective Trauma in Rwanda, *European Journal of Psychotraumatology*, 6, 10. doi:10.3402/ejpt.v6.28706

Johnstone, L. & Boyle, M. (2018). *The Power Threat Meaning Framework*. Leicester: British Psychological Society, Division of Clinical Psychology.

Kahneman, D., Slovic, P. & Tversky, A. (1982). *Judgments Under Uncertainty: Heuristics and Biases*. Cambridge: Cambridge University Press.

Lancaster, C. L., Teeters, J. B., Gros, D. F. & Back, S. E. (2016). Posttraumatic Stress Disorder: Overview of Evidence-Based Assessment and Treatment. *Journal of Clinical Medicine*, 5 (11), 105.

Laville, S. (Thursday 11 February2016). Hogan-Howe Criticised for Comments Regarding Child Sex Abuse Claims. *The Guardian*.

Mannarino, A. P., Cohen, J. A., Deblinger, E., Runyon, M. K. & Steer R. A. (2012). Trauma-Focused Cognitive-Behavioral Therapy for Children Sustained Impact of Treatment 6 and 12 Months Later. *Child Maltreatment*, 17 (3), 231–241.

Masson, J. M. (1984). *The Assault on Truth: Freud's Suppression of the Seduction Theory*. London: Penguin.

McGlynn, C. & Westmarland, N. (2019). Kaleidoscopic Justice: Sexual Violence and Victim-Survivors' Perceptions of Justice. *Social & Legal Studies*, 28 (2), 179–201.

Mehta, J., Clifford, E., Taggart, D. and Speed, E. (2017). "Where Your Mental Health Disappears Overnight": Disabled People's Experiences of the Employment and Support Allowance Work Related Activity Group. London: Inclusion London.

McDonagh, F. (2009). *Dom Helder Camara: Essential Writings*. New York: Orbis Books.

Million, D. (2013). *Therapeutic Nations*. Arizona: University of Arizona Press.

Munro, E. (1996). Avoidable and Unavoidable Mistakes in Child Protection. *British Journal of Social Work*, 26, 793–808.

Munro, E. (1999). Common Errors of Reasoning in Child Protection Work. *Child Abuse & Neglect*, 23, 745–758.

NHS Scotland. (2017). *Transforming Psychological Trauma: A Knowledge and Skills Framework for the Scottish Workforce*. Edinburgh: NHS Education for Scotland.

O'Neill, A., Sojo, V., Fileborn, B., Scovelle, A. J. & Milner, A. (2018). The #MeToo Movement: An Opportunity in Public Health? *The Lancet*, 391, 2587–2588.

Orwell, G. (1949). *1984*. London: Penguin.

Peake, A. & Fletcher, M. (1997). *Strong Mothers: A Resource for Mothers of Children Who Have Been Sexually Assaulted*. Lyme Regis: Russell House Publishing.

Pearce, W. B. & Cronen, V. E. (1980). *Communication, Action and Meaning: The Creation of Social Realities*. New York: Praeger.

Read, J., Hammersley, P. & Rudegeair, T. (2007). Why, When and How to Ask About Child Abuse. *Advances in Psychiatric Treatment*, 13, 101–110.

Reason, J. (1998). Achieving a Safe Culture: Theory and Practice. *Work & Stress*, 12 (3), 293–306.

Reason, J. (2000). Human Error: Models and Management. *British Medical Journal*, 320, 768–770.

Rouf, K. & Rhodes, E. (2017). Revealing Hidden Issues. *The Psychologist*, 30. https://thepsychologist.bps.org.uk/volume-30/november-2017/revealing-hidden-issues.

Rouf, K. (1989). Journey Through Darkness: The Path from Victim to Survivor. *Child Sexual Abuse, DECP Occasional Papers*, 6 (1), 6–10.

Rouf, K. (1990). Myself in echoes: my voice in song. In A. Bannister, K. Barrett & E. Shearer (Eds.), *Listening to Children: The Professional Response to Hearing the Abused Child*. Essex: Longman.

Rouf, K. & Taggart, D. (5 September2018) Is There Justice for Trauma Survivors? *Cost of Living blog*. https://www.cost-ofliving.net/is-there-justice-for-trauma-survivors/

Spicer, D. (2018). *Joint Serious Case Review Concerning Sexual Exploitation of Children and Adults with Needs for Care and Support in Newcastle-upon-Tyne*. Newcastle: Safeguarding Children's Board and Newcastle Safeguarding Adults Board.

Smail, D. (2005). *Power, Interest and Psychology: Elements of a Social-Materialist Understanding of Distress*. London: PCCS Books.

Sweeney, A.Clement, S.Filson, B. & Kennedy, A. (2016). Trauma-Informed Mental Healthcare in the UK: What is It and How Can We Further Its Development? *Mental Health Review Journal*, 21 (3), 174–192.

Taggart, D. (2016). Notes from the Underground: Some Reflections on Clinical Psychology's Role in Responding to Historical and Institutional Child Sexual Abuse. *Clinical Psychology Forum*, 286.

Taggart, D. (2017). Anatomised. *Asylum Magazine for Democratic Psychiatry, 24* (1).

Sweeney, A. & Taggart, D. (2018). (Mis)understanding Trauma-Informed Approaches in Mental Health. *Journal of Mental Health*. doi:10.1080/09638237.2018.1520973

Taggart, D. & Speed, E. (2019). Stigma and Mental Health: Exploring Potential Models to Enhance Opportunities for a Parity of Participation. *Journal of Ethics in Mental Health*, 10 (VI).

Tajfel, H. & Turner, J. C. (1979). An Integrative Theory of Intergroup Conflict. In W. G. Austin & S. Worchel (Eds.), *The Social Psychology of Intergroup Relations*. Monterey, CA: Brooks/Cole, pp. 33–47.

Tajfel, H. & Turner, J. C. (1986). The Social Identity Theory of Inter-Group Behavior. In S. Worchel and L. W. Austin (Eds.), *Psychology of Intergroup Relations*. Chicago: Nelson-Hall.

Taylor, K. (2004). *Brainwashing*. Oxford: Oxford University Press.

Thibodeau, R., Kim, S. & Jorgensen, R. S. (2011). Internal Shame, External Shame, and Depressive Symptoms: A Meta-Analytic Review. *Psychology Faculty Publications*, 4. http://fisherpub.sjfc.edu/psychology_facpub/4.

United Nations. (1989). *Convention on the Rights of the Child*. Geneva: United Nations [retrieved on 26 February 2018]. http://www.ohchr.org/en/professionalinterest/pages/crc.aspx.

United Nations. (2015). *Transforming our World: the 2030 Agenda for Sustainable Development*. Geneva: United Nations. https://www.un.org/ga/search/view_doc.asp?symbol=A/RES/70/1&Lang=E

Waites, B. & Rouf, K. (2014). Reflections from the Front Line: Safeguarding Children and Helping Adults Who Disclose Historical Abuse. *Clinical Psychology Forum*, 262, 40–43.

Walker, P. (Sunday 10 February2013). Frances Andrade Killed Herself After Being Accused of Lying, Says Husband. *The Guardian*.

Wright, K. (2018). Challenging Institutional Denial: Psychological Discourse, Therapeutic Culture and Public Inquiries. *Journal of Australian Studies*, 42 (2), 177–190. doi:10.1080/14443058.2018.1462237.

Yeats, W. B. (2000). *The Second Coming. Selected Poems*. London: Penguin Modern Classics.

Zimbardo, P. G. (2007). *The Lucifer Effect: How Good People Turn Evil*. New York: Rider.

Acknowledgments

The authors take responsibility for their work, but wish to acknowledge and thank Lisa Ward, Chief Executive Officer, Oxfordshire Sexual Abuse and Rape Crisis Centre; Peter Saunders; Dr Jon Bird, Head of Research Analysis, NAPAC; Duncan Craig, Chief Executive Officer and Trauma – Focused Therapist, Manchester Survivors. We are grateful for their comments and discussions in the preparation of this chapter.

The views expressed in this chapter are our own.

Part 2.

Proposed guidelines for a code of ethical conduct for engaging with victims and survivors

It is proposed that victims and survivors of abuse should have access to a unified code of ethics to ensure that institutions, disciplines and professionals respond in ways which respect survivors' autonomy, privacy, dignity, best interests, rights to just treatment and avoidance of harm.

Such a code would also meaningfully engage in professional reflection and continuous learning, in order to flatten professional power, decolonize practice and to ensure equitable access to help. This would centralise social justice.

Such a document would not be designed to replace any existing individual codes of professional practice, but to enhance what is available and to address the particular issues faced by victims and survivors.

We call for such a code to be co-produced with victims and survivors, including those from under-served communities. We call for it to be a "living document", which should be freely available and accessible to survivors, and shared with them routinely as they access any services from which they need help, be that healthcare, social care, the police or legal system.

Some proposed ideas are laid out below:

Survivors of abuse should have the

- right to feel confident that disclosures will be taken seriously
- right to be treated in line with Equality Law
- right to question their treatment if needed
- right to be heard and respected
- right to help and to be meaningfully included in how that help is structured within the system (co-produced, trauma informed services)
- right to justice (both social and legal)
- right to see someone who has been trained and is competent in trauma informed approaches
- right to appropriate and timely support in the aftermath of abuse
- right to a textured discussion about how to respond to safeguarding concerns, unless there are accountable reasons why that cannot take place
- right to evidence based approaches, but also pluralism of approach to reflect the diverse nature of those who have been abused – there should be fidelity to following principles across approaches. These principles should focus on empowerment; support; empathy; validation; acknowledgement; normalising; understanding; personal engagement and connection

In training – trainees should have access to narratives and understandings which are informed by victims and survivors; they should be encouraged to engage critically with past and current theories about abuse; they should be aware of societal level reactions towards abuse and the stereotypes, heuristics and power dynamics which can impact on decision-making in clinical work.

In research – research should be reflective and ethical in nature; researchers should be aware of how social context, stereotypes, heuristics and power dynamics can be implicit within research agenda. Survivors should be made aware that even those research questions which are asked, and how research is funded (or not) can be subject to heuristics and biases. Researchers need to be clear and transparent about the scope of the work they have conducted; the parameters and limitations of what has been learnt; the potential applications to other settings; and also be transparent and clear about the gaps in understanding of phenomena. Victims and survivors should be invited and engaged to provide a triangulated view of research, to participate in critiquing research findings and invited to comment on applications which may affect their treatment in any domain.

In clinical settings and outside the therapy setting

- **Clinicians need to be trauma informed** – to understand the huge normative pressures on victims not to tell, to understand the years of silencing that may occur as a result not only of the abuser's individual attempts to silence and isolate victims, but also the huge societal narratives which question and blame victims and how these narratives can become internalized by victims and silence them further. Clinicians need to have good understandings of trauma and its impacts on the individual and their attachment relationships.

- **Clinicians need to be reflective** – clinicians are as vulnerable to hidden or Grand Narratives as any other person as they are embedded within history and still appear in contemporary society. It is important to reflect on these and to ensure that unhelpful biases against survivors are discussed in supervision.

- **Clinicians can help to change perceptions** – clinicians have a role to play in preventing the 'othering' of survivors. The shared aim of stopping abuse, preventing abuse and supporting survivors means that societal structures must adopt ways to embed support for them. This also suggests that the 'othering' of abusers may need to change, in order to help those who disclose abuse to be believed; to work on ways of ensuring there is restorative/ social/ legal justice for survivors and that ultimately the aim needs to be to stop abuse. Clinicians can help to formulate at an individual level, within team settings and respectfully work on helping inform the public about abuse, to ensure that work can be done at differing levels of society. This also involves working to reduce all forms of discrimination which lead to inequalities and injustices. It involves efforts to incorporate the impact of intersectionality into professional thinking, and to pay attention to hierarchies of vulnerability. It includes scrutiny and challenging power, such as expectations which promote harmful masculine identities, and highlighting how these have a toxic impact upon everyone in society.

   This also means drawing out implicit assumptions and to question them; to tackle misunderstandings around victims of abuse, to avoid their re-victimisation; to be person centred; have an understanding of social context; be committed to social action to increase public awareness of trauma and to work to prevent it.

- **Build trauma informed practice into service design** – clinicians and managers need to understand that survivors may suffer repeated harms, not only from the original experiences of abuse, but also from how others respond to them, either inadvertently or intentionally. Survivors may not get either social or legal justice. Embedded power at every level in social structures can prevent this and everyday interactions may serve to compound experiences of trauma; for example, the survivor is referred away from the therapy services repeatedly and sign-posted to other less effective sources of help. Managers need to work on co-produced service design with survivors in order to provide services that respond to the nature of their experiences and their needs. There needs to be a common commitment to the adequate funding of such services, which ultimately prevent repeated cycles of harm and suffering, and ensure a healthier community.

- **Be aware of the potential limitations of diagnosis and keep a client centred approach** – clinicians need to fully appreciate the potential limitations of diagnostic systems for people who have suffered chronic trauma. Diagnostic labels do not say anything about 'prognosis'. Many people can find it a relief to have a diagnosis, as it can remove a sense of self-blame and confusion about what is happening to them.

  However, it is important to recognise that this is not the case for everyone, and there are particular diagnoses which may be problematic, most notably, the label 'personality disorder' which can reflect embedded power. It may locate problems within the individual; does not fully appreciate the presence or impact of trauma; is suggestive of a therapeutic fatalism (as personality tends to be perceived as fixed, having a 'disorder of personality' sounds like change is not possible). In reality, it becomes shorthand which can become pejorative and a reason to stop people accessing services which are open to others. Such labels are being attached to people earlier and earlier (there are examples of young people in CAMHS services being told that they have "an emerging personality disorder").

  Such personality based diagnoses, may also be unhelpful for staff – for instance, the term 'personality disorder' can act as a hook upon which to put their own understandable stresses, when working in systems that are not trauma informed in approach. Working with traumatized survivors can lead to secondary trauma for clinicians, because therapy can be stressful and challenging (as well as rewarding and vocational).

- **Services must design-in staff wellbeing** – following on from the above point, services must be designed to support those who work with people who are traumatized so they are protected from secondary harm, and so that they can respond in helpful ways to survivors (e.g. taking disclosures seriously and ensuring other children are protected from harm).

- **Therapeutic approaches** – offers of help should be holistic and not operate in ways that recreate trauma responses; be evidence based but aware of the limits of the evidence base, and to commit to evidence based practice; be pluralistic; acknowledge that abuse is based in interpersonal harm and so healing can come from experiencing healthy interpersonal processes. Restorative healing may go beyond traditional notions of therapy, and also involve connection or reconnection with activities and communities that restore hope, meaning, creativity and a sense of purpose or social action.

Index

Note: **bold** page numbers indicate tables.

Milton Keynes UK
Ingram Content Group UK Ltd.
UKHW022034130923
428635UK00013B/69

9 781032 044293